Getting to Healthy

Also by John S. Hoffman, Ph.D.

Surviving Driving: What Every New Driver Should Know Before Getting Behind the Wheel

The Emotional Foundations of Loving Relationships

Instructional Design: Step by Step

Instructional Development: Step by Step

Getting to Healthy

Making the Transition to Eating Real Food

John S. Hoffman, Ph.D.

This book contains health information and motivational advice intended to prompt the reader to eat a healthier diet. This book is not intended as a substitute for medical advice from your physician or other trained health professional. The reader should consult a physician or other trained medical health professional in all matters regarding his or her health and before changing his or her diet or starting any program or treatment. Although every effort has been made to ensure the accuracy of the information in this book at the time it was published, there may be mistakes, both typographical and in content. The publisher and the author disclaim liability for any medical outcomes or adverse effects that may occur as a result of following the advice or methods suggested in this book.

Getting to Healthy: Making the Transition to Eating Real Food

Copyright © 2019 John S. Hoffman

All rights reserved. No part of this book may be used or reproduced by any means, graphic, electronic, or mechanical, including photocopying, recording, taping or by any information storage retrieval system without the written permission of the publisher except in the case of brief quotations embodied in critical articles and reviews.

ISBN: 978-1-7944-3297-0

Cover photo by Shutterstock

*To my wife
for helping me in my journey
to get to healthy*

CONTENTS

Part 1. Why Make the Change?	1
Part 2. Twenty-One Weeks of Daily Motivation	13

Week 1
The healthiest diet on the planet	17
Race horse or junk heap?	18
The diet recommended by the largest U.S. managed health care organization	19
Does how you eat determine how you will die?	20
Have we made a deal with the nutritional devil?	20
A powerful strategy for eating healthier	21
Some immediate benefits from healthy eating	22

Week 2
Ten easy things you can do right now to eat healthier	25
The lottery you are guaranteed to win	26
Trying to eat healthier? Strive for progress, not perfection	28
Why are foods like pizza, burgers, and chocolate chip cookies so addictive?	28
Want to know why healthy eating is important? Watch this!	29
Turning a blind eye to mounting scientific evidence	30
Understanding consequences before making choices	31

Week 3
Will your friends pay for *your* poor dietary choices?	37
Escaping the pleasure trap: Part 1	38
Escaping the pleasure trap: Part 2	39
Escaping the pleasure trap: Part 3	41
Escaping the pleasure trap: Part 4	43
What you leave behind when you stop eating junk food	47
Is healthy eating extreme?	48

Week 4
About the "Aligning the stars in your favor" series	53
Aligning the stars in your favor: Controlling your food environment	53
Aligning the stars in your favor: The power of routines	55
Aligning the stars in your favor: Making deposits into your Personal Health Account (PHA)	56
Aligning the stars in your favor: Combating emotional eating	57
Aligning the stars in your favor: Making swift course corrections	58
Aligning the stars in your favor: Taming your sweet tooth	58

Aligning the stars in your favor: Avoiding wandering eyes in the grocery store ... 60

Week 5
Aligning the stars in your favor: Changing your concept of "What is food?" ... 63
Aligning the stars in your favor: Choosing to like healthy foods ... 64
Aligning the stars in your favor: Building emotional and social support structures ... 65
Aligning the stars in your favor: Avoiding one-way doors ... 66
Aligning the stars in your favor: Treating your body with respect ... 68
Aligning the stars in your favor: Avoiding the need for medical care ... 69
Aligning the stars in your favor: Getting over your fear of eating fruits ... 70

Week 6
Are you on track for a serious train wreck? ... 75
We are not carnivorous apes ... 75
What's wrong with my mirror? ... 76
Size matters ... 76
Eat more, weigh less ... 77
What you should feed your gut flora ... 78
What is good nutrition? ... 79

Week 7
What does "zero sugar" really mean? ... 83
Are chips labeled as "veggie chips" really made from veggies? ... 83
Who's watching out for the health of our children? ... 84
What's a medium French fry worth? ... 86
Wake up, America ... 86
Diagnosis: "Unknown" ... 88
An intervention with zero side effects ... 89

Week 8
Fast food marketers strike again ... 93
The price of modern convenience ... 94
Have it your way ... 95
Americans now have almost constantly elevated insulin levels ... 96
Another example of a marketing slight-of-hand ... 97
Losing weight is not the goal ... 98
Are fast food coupons really a bargain? ... 98

Week 9
The profession unlikely to go the way of the buggy whip maker ... 103
The eat-all-you-want diet in which people lose weight ... 103

Why taking a vitamin B-12 supplement is critical for those who don't eat animal products	104
Is sweet potato the latest fad in crackers and chips?	105
Developing a deeper appreciation for natural, whole foods	106
Why you should eat breakfast at home	107
Is your body slated for "planned obsolescence"?	108

Week 10

Why you want the last years of your life to be some of your healthiest	111
Is your goal to feed your family or nourish your family?	112
Don't be afraid to learn about healthy eating	113
Firefighter satisfaction survey	114
Plant-based foods power arduous summer hike	115
The importance of eating dark, leafy greens every day	115
When the scientific universe collides with popular culture	116

Week 11

Who is cherry picking now?	121
What neglecting your health can potentially cost you	121
"Your kids will love it!"	122
The ten most addictive foods in the world (duh!)	123
Define your diet by what you eat, not by what you can't eat	124
Another reason to consider giving up eating meat: Meat may contain banned drugs	126
Where the good stuff isn't	127

Week 12

Want to slow down how fast you age?	131
Why don't people act when they know an impending disaster is coming their way?	131
When is a good time to have a heart attack?	133
Why you may want to close your kitchen early every day	134
"Life is too short not to enjoy it."	135
The problem with diets that have built-in cheat days and cheat foods	136
Can you have type 2 diabetes and not even know it?	137

Week 13

"Eating right is self-care, not deprivation"	141
Where is your "happy place"?	141
What kind of diet do your kids really eat?	142
Make it easy for your loved ones to eat healthily	144
Farsightedness may be the key to long-term health	145
More parents are taking their kids to fast-food restaurants	146
Another fast-food brand gets a makeover	147

Week 14
- Should you eat plants or jellyfish to keep your brain healthy? ... 151
- Is it good to eat like a king? ... 152
- Food that is not food. ... 152
- Does dieting lead to permanent weight loss? ... 153
- What you don't know about micronutrients can kill you ... 155
- Take a pizza, doughnut, or burger break ... 157
- A recipe for stuffed candy corn pizza—are you kidding? ... 158

Week 15
- Learning to sing ... 163
- Do you worry about your health as much as you worry about your mortgage? ... 165
- The dangers of "recreational" eating ... 165
- Another fast-food restaurant announces a customer loyalty program ... 166
- Junk food under the nutritional microscope ... 167
- Can you outrun your fork? ... 168
- Have car, will travel—and eat! ... 169

Week 16
- "Who cares if I die a few years earlier?" ... 173
- How one company encourages healthier eating on-the-job ... 174
- Understanding your daily vulnerability cycle ... 176
- Is healthy food bare, naked food? ... 178
- Your last defense ... 179
- Another fast-food distribution channel extends its reach ... 180
- Can the culture you were born into kill you? ... 181

Week 17
- Let not thy tongue be thy guide ... 185
- Does how you eat affect our environment and our planet? ... 186
- Watch out for all that extra food you eat at work ... 186
- Another upcoming fast food trend ... 187
- Avoiding medical insurance nightmares ... 188
- Salt—the other "white stuff" ... 190
- Does eating healthily build a strong immune system? ... 191

Week 18
- "This is to die for" ... 195
- Being penny wise and pound foolish ... 195
- Do we practice "healthcare" or "sickcare" in the U.S.? ... 196
- Can we exercise our way out of the obesity crisis? ... 198
- Dress for success ... 199
- Ignoring the legal fine print ... 199
- How valuable is your health? ... 200

Week 19
- Does misery motivate change? ... 205
- Make your home a "safe house" for healthy living ... 206
- Living free of food addictions ... 207
- How healthy eating becomes self-motivating ... 208
- "Fan food—not fast food" ... 209
- Are plant-based diets the nutritional equivalent of quitting smoking? ... 210
- You are in truth what you eat ... 212

Week 20
- Going nuts over nuts ... 217
- Garbage collection day for your cells ... 218
- Is what you see what you get? ... 219
- The lowdown on antioxidant-laden legumes ... 220
- Weight-loss drug brags about losing one negative side effect ... 221
- Meatless burgers ... 222
- Which organs of your body do you want to keep? ... 223

Week 21
- Is trial-and-error all you need to guide your life? ... 227
- Get moving ... 228
- Is "clean" food healthy food? ... 228
- Are you too busy to take care of your body? ... 229
- How many ways are there to justify buying and eating junk food? ... 230
- Are you conscious of just how vulnerable your body is? ... 231
- How "getting to healthy" will help you in other areas of your life ... 232

Part 3. Conclusion ... 235

About the author ... 239

PART 1.

WHY MAKE THE CHANGE?

Nine years ago, I went in to see my doctor for my annual physical examination. He noticed that my PSA test score had been steadily rising over the last few years and was starting to rise above normal. So he referred me to a urologist. Fortunately for me, the first thing the urologist did was give me a physical examination. As he did, his countenance suddenly fell, and he immediately ordered an ultrasound. The images showed a large tumor inside my left testicle. He announced that I probably had testicular cancer and would need an operation to remove the testicle.

A few days later, another technician did a painful biopsy on my prostate gland (the original reason I went to see the urologist) in which ten needles were shot through the wall of my rectum and into my prostate. The results from this biopsy showed that I had cancer in at least 30 percent of my prostate.

Being diagnosed with two different forms of deadly cancer within a two week period left me numb and in shock. I weighed 45 pounds more than my ideal weight, but otherwise considered myself healthy. I was aware of no genetic history of testicular cancer in my family. I thought I was too young to be diagnosed with two different cancers. Although my children were grown and out of the house, I wanted to see their lives unfold and have a grandfatherly influence on my grandchildren. I did not want to die.

Over the next couple of months, the surgeons removed the cancerous organs. First I had a radical inguinal orchiectomy to remove the testicle with the tumor. After the operation, the lab confirmed that the tumor was indeed testicular cancer. After letting my body heal for two months, the surgeons performed a radical prostatectomy in which my entire prostate was surgically removed along with the prostatic urethra—the section of the urethra that goes through the prostate—and some other related tissues. Of necessity, some of the nerves that serve the reproductive system were also cut, damaged, or removed. The surgery kept me bedridden for several days and away from my job for six weeks. It also left me with permanent urinary leakage and other disabilities. These were life-altering consequences.

My oncologist urged me to undergo radiation treatments to "kill off any remaining cancer cells," even though subsequent scans and tests showed no evidence that the cancer had metastasized or spread. After talking to a friend who underwent radiation treatments for his cancer, I decided to take my chances without it.

Instead, I started reading all the books and information I could on cancer. I immediately stopped eating refined carbohydrates and any food that had added sugar in it. I ate more vegetables. I quit eating all dairy and severely restricted my intake of meat. I started drinking herbal Essiac tea every day. I tried to manage stress and get adequate sleep. I took special supplements.

Unfortunately, the information that is so widely available today on nutritional research was not well known at that time or as freely available on the internet as it is today. A good deal of ground-breaking nutritional research had yet to be conducted.

For me, my surgeries and cancer diagnoses were a giant wake-up call and my first experience with one-way doors (irreversible health consequences). I had just lost one organ and one gland of my body along with their corresponding bodily functions and had been left scarred and permanently maimed. My life would be forever different from that point forward, and there was no getting that organ and gland back. For the next several years, I lived in fear of recurrence from these two cancers, wondering if I would hear a third death sentence pronounced on me at any moment—and I hadn't even committed a crime.

I couldn't help wondering why someone as healthy as I was would come down with cancer in the first place. I was only in my mid-fifties. When I asked my doctors, I couldn't get a satisfactory answer. Some said that it might be genetics or exposure to environmental toxins, some said it was just something that can happen when you "get old," and others admitted that they didn't know. All the medical establishment could do was offer me their standard medical protocols for treating cancer—surgery, chemotherapy, and radiation. I knew that the latter two treatments had limited research to back up their *long*-term effectiveness.

Unfortunately, after a few years of regular follow up exams, scans, and tests that consistently detected no further cancer, I relaxed and gradually fell back into my previous eating habits. I started eating the standard American diet (SAD) once again, buying highly processed foods at the grocery store, dining out at restaurants and fast-food establishments, and eating whatever I wanted. I was headed for another major health disaster, *and I didn't even know it*.

But I should have known better. Intuition alone should have told me that I could not expect my body to kill off existing cancer cells and fight off new diseases if I fed it a diet of nutrient-deficient fast foods, processed foods, and junk foods. After all, who really believes that the fine powder that comes out of a cake mix box is good for you? It wasn't until later, after I gained a deeper understanding of healthy eating, that I understood *why* the food I was eating would lead me through more one-way doors.

Then one day, I happened to switch on a television talk show in which guest Dr. Joel Fuhrman was talking about his newest book, which, at that time, was *The End of Dieting*. I listened intently. What I heard made a lot of sense. His advice to stop chasing after the latest diet and instead just eat the healthiest, most nutrient-dense whole foods for the rest of my life rang true. All the research he quoted and the benefits he recited further piqued my interest. I immediately ordered his book.

That small decision was a turning point in my life and marked the beginning of my quest to learn more about healthy eating. I shared what I heard with my wife, and she also became interested. Over the next year and a half, we implemented changes to our diet, eating more fruits and vegetables; dark-green leafy salads; intact grains such as brown rice, steel-cut oats, and quinoa; cooked mushrooms; 100 percent whole wheat bread made from scratch; beans and other legumes; and raw, unsalted nuts and seeds. I also stopped eating meat, most dairy, and eggs (my wife had already stopped eating these things previously).

But that is where I plateaued. I was addicted to certain junk foods such as ice cream, pizza, chocolate chip cookies, cake, donuts, buttered popcorn, and chips. I used these foods like a magic wand to self-soothe at the end of the day, as an emotional crutch when I was feeling down, and to entertain my palate when I was relaxing in front of the television. For a long time, I didn't even believe I would be able to give them up. These foods were one of my few remaining pleasures in life. Or so I thought.

It was only through an intense study of healthy eating that I finally accepted the overwhelming evidence that junk food was not just nutritionally deficient, but harmful to my body. I read books like Dr. Fuhrman's *Fast Food Genocide: How Processed Food Is Killing Us and What We Can Do About It*, Dr. Michael Greger's *How Not to Die: Discover the Foods Scientifically Proven to Prevent and Reverse Disease*, Rip Esselstyn's *My Beef with Meat: The Healthiest Argument for Eating a Plant-Strong Diet*, and Douglas Lisle and Alan Goldhamer's *The Pleasure Trap: Mastering the Hidden Force that Undermines Health & Happiness*. I visited websites, read articles, watched videos, and saw outstanding documentaries on healthy eating like *Food Choices*, *Forks Over Knives*, *Fed Up*, and *What the Health* (on Netflix at the time). I couldn't deny what I had learned. I knew I had to change.

But giving up addictive, pleasurable junk foods wasn't easy. I didn't succeed on my first, second, or even my twentieth attempt. I went through withdrawal multiple times whenever I tried to give them up and suffered repeated relapses. I tried some things that failed and other things that helped. It took well over a year of persistent, determined effort to finally go completely "clean."

But it was worth it. Miraculous things started to occur with my health. I lost 45 pounds with very little effort and went down seven inches in waist size. Many of my minor health issues cleared up. My total cholesterol, which had been high, dropped below 150, with outstanding LDL, HDL, and triglyceride numbers. My blood pressure dropped to levels I hadn't seen since I was in my twenties. My energy levels increased, and over the summer, I climbed numerous challenging 11,000-foot to 12,000-foot mountains all summer long with outstanding speed and endurance, even passing up some of the younger hikers on the trail. I skied my heart out all winter long. I was feeling young again.

My wife told me that I looked younger and was better looking than I had been in decades. My food cravings all but vanished. I was able to walk down the aisles of the grocery store without struggling over which junk food items I was going to buy. I developed a deep respect for my body and wanted to feed it only the best, most nutritious "fuels." I loved the way I felt. And best of all, I enjoyed all these benefits *without* expensive medications that always come with nasty side effects.

That was my saga. That is why I made the change to healthy eating. Having made the change and experienced the benefits, I now wanted to help others who were interested in doing the same. That is why I wrote this book. No matter what your level of desire to eat healthier, you can do it. So let's get started!

Before you set out on your quest, however, you should know that getting to healthy is a journey that requires significant planning and preparation. It is not a one-time event. Rather, it is like planning to climb a high mountain peak. First, you need information on how to prepare for the climb and what to take. Then, you need maps or an experienced guide to lead the way who is familiar with the challenges and obstacles you will encounter and how to surmount them. Then, you need to acquire the proper equipment and clothing. Next, you need to get into shape by building up your legs and your cardiovascular endurance. And finally, if you didn't secure a guide, you need others to go along with you for companionship, support, and safety.

Getting to healthy has similar requirements. First, you must be convinced that climbing the mountain is a good thing to do. You must really want the benefits for yourself. Second, you must study the map, which is a knowledge of three things: nutritional cause-and-effect relationships, which foods you should and shouldn't eat, and why. Unless you know your map, you might end up marooned on some high cliffs, suffer a fall, get lost, or otherwise have to be rescued. Understanding why you should make the climb and knowing the path to follow are both addressed through nutritional education.

But how can you get this education? The easiest way is to read the books, visit the websites, and watch the documentaries I just mentioned. These authors and documentary producers do a masterful job of explaining what the latest nutritional science says is the healthiest diet for humans. They also lay out the benefits you can expect and the serious consequences that follow when you just go along with the crowd.

"But wait," you say. "Aren't there are a lot of conflicting books and opinions out there on nutrition? How can I know that these authors and documentary writers are unbiased and balanced in their reporting?" Great question.

First of all, *everyone* has some bias in what they write, say, or recommend. You will be hard pressed to find *anyone* who is *completely* unbiased. Everyone is human. People look at the research and draw their own conclusions, which in turn colors how they look at additional research and what they say. Moreover, if someone is enthusiastic about a cause, they will likely have some bias in favor of it, which is not necessarily a bad thing if what they are promoting is the truth, or the best version of it that science can offer. So if you think you can find a source that is completely unbiased, you had better start looking on another planet.

Of course, there are plenty of strongly biased opinions out there. Likely candidates include individuals who have an obvious (or hidden) *financial or other stake* in what they are recommending. This is true even for organizations, institutions, corporations, and government agencies that stand to gain financially or in other ways from what they are recommending (watch the documentary, *What the Health*, to see some powerful examples).

But just because bias exists does not mean that *everyone* is equally biased. Some proponents are far less biased and far more objective than others. The question is, how can you tell who is less biased?

In my judgment, those who are less biased:

- Are not aligned with, affiliated with, or paid by an industry, agency, or commercial party that will benefit from the stated recommendations.
- Back up their overall conclusions with *thousands* of documented studies conducted by reputable institutions from around the world, including huge landmark studies that follow thousands or tens of thousands of subjects over many years.
- Have reference sections in their books that are very sizable, are broad in scope, and represent research across a wide number of highly esteemed and reputable universities and institutions.

I believe that Dr. Joel Fuhrman and Dr. Michael Greger both fall into the "less biased" category:

- They meet the three criteria I just mentioned.
- Their core recommendations are generally in line with many other recognized nutritional researchers and health advocates.
- They are quick to point out any tentative conclusions they make that are based only on limited research.
- They admit that their conclusions are not "locked into stone." They call their recommendations "evidence-based nutrition"—they go where the evidence from the latest body of research takes them, even if it means refuting or modifying statements that they previously made. While some authors rigidly stick to their original recommendations—even decades down the line when overwhelming research proves them wrong—these two leading health authorities do not.

But be forewarned. Anyone can do a quick search on the internet and find negative reviews on any noteworthy person. Those who pass judgment on the life's work of others based solely on the opinions of a few strangers who have unknown hidden agendas and axes to grind, are, by definition, highly biased themselves and shouldn't be casting stones. Better to conduct your own open-minded investigation, which requires, *at the very least*, that you read their books before you draw any conclusions.

So, how does this book fit into the picture? First, it will not in any way attempt to recreate what these other internationally recognized experts in healthy eating have already so brilliantly provided by the way of nutrition education. The purpose of this book is *not* to lay down another layer of highly documented nutritional facts or relationships, but to offer motivation and encouragement to those currently in the trenches who are trying to *change* how they eat.

For this reason, it will not reference every fact and tidbit of information that I mention that I have gathered from various reputable sources. This is a coaching book, not another treatise on nutrition. As such, it assumes that what these leading authorities recommend is indeed the best dietary advice on the planet (as I believe it is). It will simply remind readers from time to time of some of the facts, conclusions, and recommendations these sources have made when it reinforces important points.

In short, this book works in conjunction with these other foundational books, not as a replacement for them. You should study those books carefully and thoroughly as part of your overall education in healthy eating.

This book is designed to help you make the transition to healthy eating, once you have decided to do so. You may not know it now, but you will need a boatload of motivation to make it through the difficult withdrawal and recovery phases that follow your abstaining from junk food and other addictive foods. After acquiring a basic knowledge of nutrition, *motivation is the key to getting to healthy*. Without it, nutritional knowledge just sits on the shelf and collects dust while potential health benefits are thrown away. But motivation has a very short half-life. It must be renewed on a daily basis. Hence this book.

You are surrounded on all sides by powerful forces that threaten your desire to eat healthily. Addictive foods are found in the junk food aisles of your local grocery store, in fast food restaurants that dot every corner in every city, in neighborhood convenience stores, and even in the checkout lines of your local cloth store, where racks of candy bars stare you in the face as you wait your turn to buy a few bolts of cloth. Powerful inner drives and psychological needs also demand satisfaction through emotional, binge, and junk food eating. Finally, repeated failed attempts to give up addictive foods can take their toll on your self-esteem and self-confidence. Unless you can recharge your motivation to eat healthily every day, you will likely succumb to these powerful influences.

As one who has successfully scaled the mountain, I know where many of the dead-end trails and overhangs are. I have experienced what works and what doesn't work. And I have acquired certain insights and motivational tips from my formal education in psychology and from my own life experiences. All of this will help you in your journey.

You may be wondering if there is more than one trail that leads to the summit. Yes. I know of at least two heavily trafficked summit trails. The *cold-turkey trail* is one in which you "clean house" of all your junk food and give up unhealthy foods all at once, like addicts do in a twelve-step program. This approach works well for many people *if* they have made the proper preparation *and* they have adequate support and motivation through the difficult withdrawal phase.

Another popular trail is the *substitution trail* in which you gradually substitute healthy foods and dishes for unhealthy ones. Over time, the healthy foods crowd out the unhealthy foods, resulting in healthier eating. Both approaches have their advantages and disadvantages, which I discuss in this book. You can decide which approach works best for you, or you can forge your own one-of-a-kind trail.

Regardless of which trail you follow, one of the most difficult challenges you will face is successfully getting through the withdrawal phase that begins immediately after you stop eating unhealthy food. To help with this, I discuss why junk foods are addictive, overview the addiction and recovery process, and provide a detailed list of tips to help you prepare for and successfully navigate through withdrawal (see the four-part series of articles entitled, "Escaping the pleasure trap" in Part 2).

Another major challenge to getting to healthy is your fear of giving up eating pleasurable foods. Many people are not even willing to consider changing their diet for this very reason. The best way to address this fear is by proving it wrong. Plant-based recipes can taste delicious when they have the right combination of textures, spices, and flavors. Who is going to complain if you substitute one gourmet-tasting food for another? And when you have gone completely whole food, plant-based for a few weeks, your taste buds will change.

To further combat this fear, try out plant-based recipes and become proficient in preparing them. Yes, you will need to learn how to cook with unfamiliar (plant-based) ingredients, but this is easily done by following the instructions in each recipe. Look at it as an exciting adventure. Be persistent and patient. Expect some "failures" along the way (recipes you prepare that you don't like). Realize that such a large undertaking cannot be accomplished overnight. Continue your normal diet while you develop this new skill and build your new recipe collection. When you find recipes you like, substitute them in your weekly diet for less healthy meals. Give your taste buds time to

adjust to the new flavors and taste sensations. Over time, you will be successful.

Recipes can be found online on websites such as ForksOverKnives.com, DrFuhrman.com, and Engine2Diet.com and in the many vegan and plant-based recipe books, including Dr. Michael Greger's, *The How Not to Die Cookbook*. However, be aware that some "vegan" recipes call for ingredients—cooking oil, added sugar, salt, white flour, and other ingredients—that are not part of a nutritarian diet (for more information on the nutritarian diet, see the first article in Part 2 entitled, "The healthiest diet on the planet").

In Part 2 of this book, I provide daily motivational coaching. This section is divided into 21 weeks of seven short articles per week that are intended to be read daily—one per day—to strengthen your resolve to eat healthier. These 147 articles should be enough to keep you motivated all the way through withdrawal and into recovery and beyond.

How do they do this? Through the use of short stories, analogies, rehearsals of key facts and statistics, exposure of faulty logic and reasoning, an examination of our cultural norms, looking at things from a novel perspective, exposure of junk-food marketing tactics, the sharing of methods for assessing the nutritional value of a food, providing strategies for dealing with social push back, rehearsing benefits and long-term consequences, and exposing people's inner thoughts that sabotage motivation. These articles will help mold you into a powerful and cunning warrior who can lay siege against the forces of unhealthy eating.

One last insight. Getting to healthy is an ideal that is not for everyone, just as not everyone who starts an exercise routine on a treadmill will want to become a chiseled fitness trainer. While acknowledging this fact may seem out of place in a book designed to motivate people to adopt the healthiest diet in the world, people have their own health and dietary goals, which I respect. Just as there are many degrees of physical fitness, there are many degrees of healthy eating, each with its own level of reward and consequences. While this book holds up the "gold standard," it will also help those who only want to climb part way up the mountain.

For them, they just might be surprised upon reaching the rarified air high up on the mountainside to find themselves renewed, invigorated, and motivated to climb up to the next higher ridge. Healthy eating eventually becomes self-motivating as you begin to experience the amazing benefits that are almost too good to be true.

So, whatever your goals are, let's get started.

Happy hiking!

PART 2.

TWENTY-ONE WEEKS OF DAILY MOTIVATION

WEEK 1

"Let's get started."

The healthiest diet on the planet

I have tried to make the recommended food choices in this book be in sync with the *nutritarian diet*, as defined by Dr. Joel Fuhrman. The nutritarian diet is not a "diet" in the traditional sense—one you go on to lose weight. Rather, it is a *way of eating* that focuses on eating *only* nutrient-dense foods and foods that are known to prevent or reduce your chance of developing health-related diseases for the remainder of your life. I believe it is the healthiest diet on the planet.

For those who aren't familiar with this diet (which Dr. Fuhrman explains in detail in almost all of his books and on his website), I'll attempt a synopsis here. The nutritarian diet prescribes eating a *variety* of whole, plant-based foods, with special emphasis on eating the following highly nutrient-dense foods *every day*:

- A wide variety of vegetables, with generous portions of cruciferous vegetables and raw, leafy greens,
- Berries and a wide assortment of other fruits,
- Legumes, including beans, lentils, peas, and chickpeas,
- Intact grains, such as wheat berries, steel-cut oats, brown rice, and quinoa,
- Mushrooms (at least partially cooked),
- Onions,
- Raw, unroasted, unsalted nuts and seeds, such as walnuts, almonds, cashews, pecans, pistachios, flax seeds (ground up so they can be digested), chia seeds, sesame seeds, pumpkin seeds, hemp seeds, and sunflower seeds, and
- A vitamin supplement for vitamin B-12 because this vitamin is not found in plant-based sources of food.

The nutritarian diet also *excludes* the following:

- Meat (if you insist on eating meat, he says to eat it infrequently and only in very tiny portions),
- Dairy, including milk, cheese, ice cream, and yogurt,
- Eggs,
- All highly processed foods (including most packaged goods at the grocery store), especially foods containing added salt and highly processed ingredients such as cooking oil and other processed

fats, white flour, white sugar, white rice, white potatoes, white pasta, and chemical preservatives, additives, and enhancers,
- Fast food from fast food and other restaurants, and
- All commercial junk food, such as candy, chips, soda, donuts, cookies, and cake.

Because this list of exclusions goes way beyond just abstaining from animal products, his diet is *not* the same as a "vegan diet," although technically those following a nutritarian diet could be considered "vegan" if they don't eat *any* animal products. However, because you could live off of French fries, potato chips, and soda and still be considered a vegan, being a "vegan" is *not* the same as being a "nutritarian." You are a nutritarian only if you exclusively eat the *nutrient-dense* whole, plant-based foods that I just described (hence the name, "nutritarian") and avoid the "foods" in the prohibited list.

Because Dr. Michael Greger recommends a very similar diet (download his free app "Daily Dozen" from your device's app store to see what he recommends eating every day; visit his website, nutritionfacts.org; or read his book *How Not to Die*), in this book, I will consider the two in the same general category in my discussions.

Race horse or junk heap?

Recently I heard a guest psychiatrist on a TV talk show ask the following question: "Would you buy a million-dollar race horse and then feed it junk food?" He then talked about the importance of respecting your body and eating a wholesome diet, getting enough exercise, and getting adequate sleep to your overall well-being and happiness.

Our bodies are certainly more complex and valuable than a million-dollar racehorse. But many of us treat our bodies like we do our cars, thinking we can drive them into the ground, ignore proper maintenance, and then take them in to a mechanic (doctor) to be "fixed" with a few new parts (medicines) and turns of a wrench (surgical procedures). The government regulates the quality of the fuel we put into our cars, but there are no such safeguards in place for the fuel we put into our bodies. We are free to put trash into our bodies if we want to, and many people do. But we are also free to eat only real, natural foods and avoid the damaging "contaminants" found in "fake" foods.

As Dr. Joel Fuhrman, the author of numerous excellent books on nutrition, likes to say, "You cannot buy good health—you must earn it through healthy eating." In fact, the most important thing you can do with regards to what you eat is this: Prepare and eat real food. In other words, eat the foods that Mother Nature—the master engineer—designed for humans— the kind that grow from the ground that are overflowing with nutrition and unadulterated by food processing.

The diet recommended by the largest U.S. managed health care organization

What diet does Kaiser Permanente, the largest U.S. managed health care organization, recommend to their physicians and patients since 2013? A *plant-*based diet. In their online brochure, after listing the many amazing benefits of a plant-based diet (lower cholesterol, lower blood pressure, longer life, and less risk of cancer and diabetes, among others), they provide practical advice on what to eat, including which food groups to select food from, how many servings you need from each, tips to get started, a simple method of judging what to put on your plate, some menu ideas, and a quote about avoiding foods that come from factories instead of the ground. They obviously believe that a whole-food, plant-based diet produces healthier employees and patients who will save them money in the long run from fewer health claims.

Another excellent checklist of what you should eat each day is found in Dr. Michael Greger's free "Daily Dozen" app, which is available from your device's app store. This checklist shows what foods are found under each category, serving sizes, and links to short informative and motivational videos.

A whole-food, plant-based diet is no longer an obscure diet practiced only by a few radical "hippies" on the fringes of society. It is fast becoming more "mainstream" and socially desirable as people come to understand the powerful benefits that come from eating this way. No longer will eating real food be kept hidden in the closet.

Does how you eat determine how you will die?

Last summer, I gathered with some family members for dinner at a local Italian restaurant. I ordered the healthiest dish on the menu—spaghetti with marinara sauce—while the others ordered more traditional entrees that were definitely less healthy. Noticing my healthier selection, one of my siblings made a good-natured joke about it. Almost without thinking, I answered back, "If you eat like an American, you are going to die like an American."

Eating the standard American diet (SAD), which Dr. Joel Fuhrman calls the "deadly American diet," dramatically increases your chances from dying from any of the leading diseases that are killing Americans and shaves a few years off your lifespan. Understanding these relationships is critical to your motivation to start eating healthier. Therefore, you should learn what the top 15 causes of death are in the U.S. and how almost all of them are related to our diet and lifestyle. A good place to begin is by reading Dr. Michael Greger's book, *How Not to Die*, or by watching his video of the same name on his website, nutritionfacts.org.

Have we made a deal with the nutritional devil?

"I will give you fast food and other fine restaurants on every corner that serve mouth-watering fare; grocery stores that are 70 percent stocked with highly processed, tasty, easy-to-fix or just open-and-eat 'food;' dairy—milk, cream, yogurt, cheese, and ice cream—that will light up the central pleasure centers of your brain; processed meats that will satisfy the deepest carnivore within you; sugary drinks that fizzle and tingle as you sip them; and snacks and candies that can be stored in your pocket, purse, or briefcase and eaten at will. This is what I can offer you. Nice, isn't it? For all this pleasure, all I ask of you is a little money ... and, oh, I forgot to mention—your health! But no worries, you will have good health for a time, even if it is for a shorter time. But when your time comes (think of it as a long way off, when you are old anyway), I get to claim what is mine. Deal?"

As you ponder this proposition, the nutritional devil notices your indecision and whispers in your ear: "If you eat anything in moderation, you will be fine." "We don't really know for sure that the standard American diet is bad." "There is so much confusion about what a healthy diet is—who can know for sure?" "If what I am eating is so bad for me, why isn't my doctor warning me, why isn't the government putting out warning labels, and why would the processed food industry be conspiring against me?"

Suddenly, the good nutritional fairy pops up and whispers in your other ear: "Research shows that moderation does not prevent or cure anything." "There is widespread consensus among science-based nutritional researchers today on the basics of which foods are good and which foods are bad for your health." "Doctors are rewarded for and practice medicine that treats the symptoms—not the underlying causes—of diseases, and doctors have little or no training on nutrition in medical school." "The documentary *What the Health* explains why the government and industry giants are not looking after your health."

So, to whom will *you* pay heed?

A powerful strategy for eating healthier

Many people cannot make the change cold turkey to a healthier, whole-food, plant-based diet. Instead, you might try this proven technique of gradually crowding out the bad stuff with the good stuff. No big upfront commitment required!

For example, instead of having a bowl of sugar-laden cereal with cow's milk for breakfast, eat some steel-cut oats or old fashioned oatmeal with raisins and cinnamon with almond or soy milk poured on top. Instead of reaching for an unhealthy junk-food snack, grab an apple or some other piece of fresh fruit that is in season. Instead of eating a heaping bowl of ice cream at night (this was my downfall for many years), have a slice of watermelon, eat some fresh berries, or enjoy a homemade berry smoothie.

Continue this process, gradually and permanently replacing unhealthy foods with healthy foods. Add in additional fruits and vegetables, including dark leafy greens; beans and other legumes (for example, make homemade vegetable bean soup, chili, lentil tacos, or bean burritos); whole grains, such as brown rice, quinoa, whole-wheat pasta, and whole-wheat bread; raw, unsalted nuts; and whole seeds, such as pumpkin and sunflower seeds, ground flax, chia seeds, and sesame seeds. By eating more and more healthy foods, you will gradually crowd out the unhealthy foods in your diet.

This is also a good way of getting your family to accept eating healthily. Who is going to complain when you substitute a delicious vegan entrée for an unhealthy one? As long as it is delicious, you will hear few complaints. By taking this approach, you will also allow time for everyone's digestive systems to adjust to eating the additional fiber (a good thing!).

This method is a low-risk strategy that requires only modest commitment but increases your odds that you will successfully make the change to a healthier diet. Give it a try!

Some immediate benefits from healthy eating

As you start to eat healthier, notice these six benefits that you get to enjoy right away:

- Real food is full of fiber, so you get to chew and enjoy your food much longer than you do with "fake" food,
- Your body *feels better* and *functions better* when you eat real food,
- Your blood sugar will stabilize—you will avoid the extreme "highs" and "lows" that others have,
- You will have less room in your stomach for unhealthy food because healthy food is bulkier, fills up your stomach faster, and stimulates the stretch receptors in your stomach that you are full *before* you overeat,
- When your cells receive the complete nutrition they need from all the micronutrient-dense foods you are eating, your body will become thoroughly nourished and send out fewer desperate, last-ditch signals to your brain to eat calorically dense foods in an attempt to raise your blood sugar or feel better, and
- You will be less likely to "binge" on junk foods and other highly processed foods which contain chemicals, artificial flavors, and other engineered ingredients in them that make it so you "can't eat just one."

Be on the lookout for and notice these benefits. As you do, you will feel a stronger desire to continue enjoying these benefits by eating real food.

WEEK 2

"One week down already! Off to a good start."

Ten easy things you can do right now to eat healthier

Humans are fearful of the unknown and afraid of committing themselves to things that are different, unfamiliar, or to which they might not succeed. Because of this, asking people to switch over to a whole-food, plant based diet—especially without first establishing a foundation of knowledge and motivation to do so—is like asking them to step backwards off a cliff to rappel down a mountain.

Fortunately, would-be rapellers can practice their skills on safe ground before they hit the slopes to build up their confidence and learn what to expect. Likewise, you can take a few baby steps toward healthy eating that don't require an "all-or-nothing" commitment to step backward into thin air.

Even though these actions may not seem very significant individually, collectively they can add up to some major health benefits. That's because any little thing you do to eat healthier will have *some* beneficial effect, and the more you do, the greater the total benefit. So, stay on terra firma while you make the following "small" changes:

- Switch from regular milk to soy or almond milk. Both are much healthier than real milk—even if the nut milk has a few grams of added sugar (zero sugar is better, but your children may not accept it if it doesn't taste sweet like cow's milk does). Consuming dairy products has been likened to eating meat. Some say it's worse than eating meat. Both meat and dairy have been linked to serious health problems. Serve the milk chilled, just like cow's milk.
- Keep lots of fresh and frozen fruit on hand that is ready-to-eat. You can thaw frozen berries and fruit in a bowl in the microwave in seconds to serve a quick and tasty treat. Make sure everyone eats at least one piece of fresh fruit a day (such as an apple or pear) and some fresh or frozen berries. Fruits and berries are the second most nutrient-dense food on the planet (after vegetables).
- Replace white bread with 100 percent whole-grain bread. Make homemade, whole-wheat bread or rolls every couple of days with a heavy duty bread maker and wheat mill. If you don't want to make your own, buy a quality 100 percent whole-wheat, oil-free bread that has only healthy ingredients. Although milled grains

have a higher glycemic index than intact grains, you are still getting the entire package of nutrients (the complex carbohydrates, phytonutrients, wheat germ oil, vitamins, minerals, and fiber) from the whole grain into your body.

- Prepare and set out some cut-up fresh veggies (carrots, celery, snap peas, radishes, red cabbage, green cabbage, peppers, cucumbers, and so forth) at lunch and dinner and for snacks throughout the day, perhaps with a side of healthy hummus or natural peanut butter for dipping.
- Fix a steamed cruciferous vegetable to accompany dinner, such as broccoli, Brussels sprouts, cabbage, or cauliflower.
- Make steel-cut oats with cinnamon and raisins for breakfast several times a week.
- Buy raw, unroasted, unsalted nuts (such as almonds, cashews, pecans, walnuts, and pistachios) and encourage everyone to eat a handful every day. Those who eat nuts with their meals feel more satiated and eat fewer calories during the day. They are also a great source of healthy omega-3 fatty acids, minerals, and other nutrients. Of course, because they are higher in calories, don't eat more than a handful a day.
- Eat half an avocado every day or some fresh guacamole with your meal (but pass on the chips!) to help you feel satiated and provide some additional healthy fat.
- For an after-dinner treat, serve up a fruit smoothie or have some cut-up melons. For example, make a simple smoothie by blending a whole, ripe banana, some frozen fruit (such as frozen blueberries), and some cold soy or almond milk together in a high-speed blender. Add a handful of pre-washed, fresh baby spinach to the smoothie before you blend it for added nutrition.
- Eat on time. Don't delay lunch or dinner. Hunger tempts everyone to reach for a quick fix or an unhealthy junk-food snack.

The lottery you are guaranteed to win

Lottery fervor reached a fever pitch recently when the Mega Millions lottery jackpot rose to 1.6 billion (yes, billion) dollars. Every day that the jackpot increased, more people rushed out to buy a ticket, some even driving a hundred miles or more across state lines to secure a chance to win. News anchors reported the jackpot prize in amazement, and guests on talk shows speculated on how their lives would change if they won.

Of course, the odds of you personally winning the jackpot are astronomically small—CNN reported that it was 1 in 302,575,350. That's over 258 times less than your odds of being struck by lightning—1 in 1,171,000—in any given year and over 4,000 times less than your odds of being killed by an impact from an object from space *over your lifetime*. But fantasizing about how your life would change for the better and the bucket list you would check off is simply too much for many people to resist.

This made me wonder, how many of these same people ever think about their odds of getting chronic diseases and other health problems in their lifetime? If they knew what those odds were—and they are great—perhaps they would be more concerned about what they could do to tilt things in their favor rather than dreaming about winning the lottery.

Think about it. The lottery will only change the lifestyles of a small handful of winners—a minuscule speck of dust in the total numbers of people in the U.S. But if people changed what they eat, hundreds of millions of lives would be significantly changed for the better. Heart disease, cancer, stroke, and diabetes, which afflicts millions of lives annually, would be almost unheard of. Obesity rates and its associated health issues would plummet. Sick days would be greatly reduced. Healthcare costs would nose dive to unheard of levels, making healthcare more affordable for the millions of people who currently cannot afford it. The amount of unnecessary human grief and suffering due to preventable health problems, which has reached staggering proportions today, would be greatly eliminated.

Moreover, what good is winning the lottery if you die from an early heart attack or stroke, are in constant pain from cancer or some other disease, or if you lose your eyesight or your legs from complications of type 2 diabetes?

Rather than play the odds of winning that are over 4,000 times less than getting hit and killed by an impact from space, why don't you employ the odds that you *can* control—those of your own health destiny? By changing the way you eat, you can greatly reduce your chances of dying from nearly all of the top 15 causes of death in the U.S.

So, play the lottery in which you are guaranteed to win. The prize is a much healthier, more vibrant, and less pain-riddled life than the one you will otherwise live. You have nothing to lose, and everything to gain!

Trying to eat healthier? Strive for progress, not perfection

Every little bit of change you make toward healthier eating is progress, no matter how small. You should feel good about yourself when you make *any* change. Tell yourself, "Look what I did today to eat healthier. Isn't that great!"

Don't set yourself up for defeat by expecting yourself to eat *perfectly* healthy at all times—all that will do is cause discouragement when you don't achieve this standard, which in turn can lead to tearing yourself down, giving up, reverting back to old habits, or binging on less healthy alternatives. As Dr. Michael Greger likes to say, "It's not what you eat on your birthday or holidays that determines your overall health. It is what you eat day-in and day-out—the sum total of your diet."

Strive to make progress *over time* and remember that *everything* you do to eat healthier counts—even eating an apple a day makes a difference. If you have an occasional bad day and do some emotional eating, don't beat yourself up! Just go back to where you left off the next day. Unlike computer instructions that require perfect lines of code before producing a successful outcome, good health can be achieved incrementally as you replace one "bad" food with a "good" food, add one more healthy food to your diet, and avoid one more food that is unhealthy.

Why are foods like pizza, burgers, and chocolate chip cookies so addictive?

A recent news report stated that research shows that fats plus carbs trigger a *greater* pleasure response in your brain than the sum of the two do alone. The researchers reported that the *combination* of fats and carbs can overstimulate the brain's reward mechanism in the same way that drugs of abuse do. This helps explain why foods like pizza, burgers, French fries, chocolate chip cookies, and ice cream are so addictive. They trick our brain circuits into thinking we have found a goldmine of nutrition.

So, take a hard look every time you eat fast foods, junk foods, or processed foods. If they have both fat and blood-sugar-spiking carbohydrates in them (sugar, white flour, white rice, white potatoes, and so forth), then you can know that eating them will light up the addiction centers of your brain in a way that is similar to drugs of abuse. Isn't it time you recognize that these foods are addictive and make the decision to start eating healthily?

Want to know why healthy eating is important? Watch this!

Would you watch a few videos if you knew that the information in these videos would save you thousands of dollars over your lifetime in out-of-pocket healthcare costs, help you stay away from the hospital and doctor's office, circumvent many serious diseases and a premature death, and improve your overall health, energy, and vitality? Sound too good to be true, like an ad for a new-fangled exercise machine?

Think again. This is not an ad to get you to buy anything, but a plea to persuade you to eat healthier by taking advantage of some readily available educational materials.

A good way to get started is to watch the excellent documentaries that are available on healthy eating (see my list below). The information in these documentaries will help you understand why you should eat a healthier diet and will provide you some strong motivation to do so.

Be forewarned, though. Truth always has its detractors—people who have their own agendas and axes to grind, including not wanting to change their own diet or not wanting to threaten their own livelihoods. So don't trust someone else's opinion—not even mine! Draw your own conclusions after you watch these documentaries and do your own investigation. It only takes a few hours.

I highly recommend that you watch the following documentaries (check your streaming provider to see if they are available):

- *Forks Over Knives*
- *Food Choices*
- *What the Health*
- *Fed Up*

Then visit Dr. Michael Greger's website, nutritionfacts.org, and Dr. Joel Fuhrman's website, drfuhrman.com, and read a couple of their books, such as *How Not to Die*, *Fast Food Genocide*, or *The End of Dieting*.

Unfortunately, learning about nutrition is scary for some people. They don't want to hear things that cause them *cognitive dissonance*, which is an uncomfortable feeling that comes from having thoughts and/or actions that are inconsistent with each other. For example, they don't want to learn truths about nutrition that might be out-of-sync with their current lifestyle. People want to hear good news about their bad habits, not bad news about their bad habits—remember the *Time Magazine* cover story that butter was good for you?

It's also true that people have heard so much conflicting information about nutrition in the past that they do not know what or who they should believe. Because of this, they end up believing no one, ignoring any nutritional information, or just going along with the crowd, which today, means eating the standard American diet (SAD). But as I said before, if you eat like an American, you will die like an American. How could it be otherwise?

Better to be open-minded and start your own nutrition self-education today. Listen to the documentaries. Read a couple of the recommended books. Visit the websites I listed. Give ear to those who have made the transition to healthy eating and witness what it has done for them. You will be glad you did.

Turning a blind eye to mounting scientific evidence

I have met people who reject all the information on plant-based nutrition because they claim that the research reported in the peer-reviewed scientific journals is not "scientific"—meaning it does not meet the standards of a double-blind, randomized, controlled study in which one group is forced to eat a plant-based diet and another the standard American diet for many years.

Did you know that there was *no such study* done on cigarettes where one randomly chosen group was forced to smoke their whole lives while another was not, yet the government finally declared that smoking caused lung cancer? It took over 7,000 "non-gold-standard" research studies—studies that were more correlational in nature—to finally convince the Surgeon General of the U.S. that smoking was linked to cancer and heart disease. Meanwhile, millions of people needlessly died over decades while the "non-gold-standard" research piled up. Of course, the tobacco companies got rich selling the public products that killed them while denying that their products were harmful.

Is this what is happening today with the processed food industry and the meat, egg, and dairy industries? Watch Dr. Michael Greger's excellent short video, "Evidence Based Nutrition" to see why it is unreasonable to reject all of the other scientific evidence while claiming to accept only this strictest type of scientific research. Search on the title of the video on Dr. Greger's website, nutritionfacts.org.

Understanding this is important because those who don't want to change what they eat and those who have a financial interest in having you eat the standard American diet will use this argument to try to create doubt and confusion (a smokescreen) about what foods are healthy and what foods are not. Doubt and confusion undermine motivation.

Understanding consequences before making choices

In an episode of the TV series *Veronica Mars*, high school student Veronica attends a sex education class in which students are given a robotic baby that they must keep with them day and night. The robotic baby cries and demands attention just like a real baby to be fed, burped, changed, talked to, and comforted. The obvious intent of this "hands on" exercise is to get students to think twice before engaging in behavior that could ultimately lead to unwanted pregnancies.

When I took driver's education in high school, we were required to watch movies that showed the aftermath of various traffic accidents involving cars, trucks, and/or tractor-trailers. These films explicitly showed the injuries that people sustained that left them dead, mangled, or severely handicapped. The causes of these accidents were discussed in detail so students could form an association between poor driving decisions and their resulting consequences. I can still see many of these graphic images in my mind today, where they continue to influence my driving behavior.

Perhaps we need something similar to this to get us to consider the consequences of our eating choices before we make them. Perhaps we would eat differently if we watched real-life, graphic video clips of things like:

- A by-pass surgery,
- A column of rock-hard cholesterol being pulled out of an artery,
- A person struggling to deal with the aftereffects of powerful radiation treatments or poisonous chemotherapy,

- A firsthand look at a kidney ruined by chronic dietary abuse and the resulting lifelong required dialysis treatments,
- A person's change of life after suffering a partially paralyzing stroke,
- A close examination of a real liver that has fatty liver disease,
- A person managing their type 2 diabetes through constant glucose testing, insulin shots, and dietary restrictions,
- An Alzheimer's patient suffering progressive mental deterioration,
- The arteries of a teenager killed in an auto accident that already show significant signs of atherosclerosis ("hardening of the arteries"), and
- A documentary of how one's life is changed after suffering a serious disease or illness.

These real-life graphic examples would then be followed by frank discussions of common diseases, how they can be prevented, and the odds of contracting them if people continue to eat the standard American diet.

Some might say that such an approach would be cruel or insensitive or that it employs "scare tactics" to try to modify behavior. They argue that using "fear" to motivate people does not work in the long run. But are these really scare tactics?

Scare tactics are when people exaggerate, lie, or blow out of proportion the risks or consequences that are associated with a behavior or decision for manipulative purposes (many political ads do this). On the other hand, showing people in a calm, tactful way the *actual* and *natural consequences* that follow (or are likely to follow) certain decisions or behaviors is actually a manifestation of compassion and responsible adult behavior. It is manipulative and deceptive to *hide* the life-altering, natural consequences that follow certain destructive decisions or behaviors, such as unhealthy eating. Many who are invested in the current status quo want to do just that for financial gain.

Moreover, doesn't education consist of teaching people cause-and-effect relationships? Isn't this how we go out and effect changes in the world after we leave school? If some of these consequences are inherently "scary"—such as falling off a cliff after going around a guard rail to get a better photograph on the rim of the Grand Canyon or trying to cross a busy highway outside of a crosswalk with a traffic light—that is just the way real life is. Safety officers on an aircraft carrier do not coddle and downplay the serious consequences of unsafe flight-deck practices. Neither should we.

Of course, we should teach health-related cause-and-effect relationships at a level that is appropriate to the age, maturity, and emotional capabilities of students, but as they approach adulthood, they should be taught these relationships more fully and completely. Good health is built on knowledge—not ignorance.

WEEK 3

"You're doing great!"

Will your friends pay for *your* poor dietary choices?

One of the reasons people are reluctant to change their diet is because they are afraid of what their friends and others in their social circles will say or think of them when they turn down "socially acceptable" foods. "Let's go get a pizza for lunch." "How about coming over for a BBQ tomorrow?" "I made some special treats for you just for this occasion." People don't want to offend or lose their friends, be seen as breaking tradition, or be labeled as "weird" or "strange." So they don't say a thing.

But there is an alternative. Tell your friends that one of your new resolutions this year is to eat healthier and lose a few pounds (who can complain about that?), so you are cutting back on animal products (meat, dairy, eggs), sugar, and highly processed foods and are eating more whole fruits, vegetables, beans, whole grains, nuts, and seeds. If you like, you can mention that news stories and even popular consumer magazines are reporting that eating this way will improve your health, help you avoid disease, and increase your lifespan. Tell them that you are getting more concerned about your health as you grow older. All true statements.

You don't have to lead them on to think you have "crossed over" to the dark side to become a fanatical or militant vegan or nutritarian. You haven't, and, in fact, you should never become fanatical or militant about your food choices. This isn't a religion or a country—just a healthier way of eating. Always show respect for the food choices of others. Never give the impression that you are putting yourself on a high pedestal for "eating healthier than others." Rather, be humble and stick to the fact that you are simply trying to take care of your own health. Others are free to do what they want.

If you feel uncomfortable turning down the foods your friends offer, don't. Just eat smaller portions of the unhealthy food and larger portions of the healthy foods (usually, the salad, fruits, and vegetables). Once they see that you are serious about eating healthier, they may even start to make accommodations in what they offer you on future occasions. You can offer to bring a healthy salad, side dish, or some 100 percent whole wheat rolls with you when you are invited over. And when you go out to eat, choose the healthiest options on the menu if you can.

Over time, your friends and others will understand that you are trying to eat healthily for some pretty sound reasons, and they will respect you for that. They may even start to eat a few healthier foods in their own diet as a result of your example.

Escaping the pleasure trap: Part 1

While driving down the street the other day, a bakery catering truck turned in front of me that had an ad painted on its side that read, "You know you want one," along with a large picture of a delicious-looking brownie. My immediate reaction was "Of course I want one," but I have learned by reading *The Pleasure Trap*, by Douglas Lisle and Alan Goldhamer, that our modern world is full of artificially created, intensely pleasurable "fake foods" that tempt us at every turn with the promise of instant pleasure, but which deceive our built-in motivational mechanisms that would otherwise guide us into eating natural, healthy foods.

According to the authors, all animals, including humans, have a three-part motivational system that encourages us to seek pleasure, avoid pain, and conserve energy. At the center stage is pleasure, which rewards us for achieving important biological goals for survival and reproduction. In humans, intense pleasure comes from the release of dopamine in the pleasure centers of the brain.

Because our brain cannot sustain intense pleasure continuously, a secondary built-in motivational system also helps guide us toward our biological goals. It relies more heavily on the release of serotonin and other mood-altering chemicals in the brain. It is why "falling in love" with someone feels so good.

In the natural world, these built-in mechanisms do their job in guiding behavior toward important biological goals. However, when you alter the natural world and provide choices that are not normally available that short-circuit our means to pleasure but are ultimately self-destructive, our built-in motivational systems are deceived. Pleasure is no longer a reliable compass as to what is in our best interest. In short, we can pursue self-destructive behaviors while feeling good about it and being unaware of—or in denial of—their ultimate consequences. This is called "the pleasure trap."

For example, humans invented harmful drugs of abuse which produce intensely pleasurable experiences which deceive us into thinking that something wonderful is happening, but these feelings are deceptive. They ultimately lead to addiction and self-destructive ends. Our motivational systems were not designed to deal with these deceptive stimuli.

Because we have altered our environment so that the experience of pleasure is no longer reliable as to what is in the best interest of the person, people can do self-destructive things and feel like they are doing the right things. These unnatural stimuli play upon our motivational instincts, but they rob us of health and happiness.

Now, let's fast forward to the 21st Century. Today, we have a food landscape that is littered with addictive, artificially created stimuli—fast foods, candies, chips, ice cream, and other highly processed foods—that are designed to hijack your instincts and deceive you into thinking you are achieving biological success (pleasure) because they taste and feel good while you eat them, but unbeknownst to you, are secretly undermining your health. Our natural instinct to do what feels good has failed us.

Escaping the pleasure trap: Part 2

In my previous article, I described what Douglas Lisle and Alan Goldhamer dubbed "the pleasure trap" which describes how our built-in motivational mechanisms are deceived into thinking something is good for us because it feels good, when it may, in fact, be self-destructive. For example, highly addictive junk foods deceive our senses into thinking we have found a nutritional gold mine by spiking dopamine levels in our brains, while the consumption of these foods secretly undermines our health.

In today's society, we have all likely been repeated victims of the pleasure trap. If so, how can we escape its clutches? Our health and our lives hang in the balance. The answer is not trivial and requires a somewhat lengthy, multi-part explanation.

The first step for escaping the pleasure trap is self-education—learning how our natural instincts can be deceived so we can recognize when it is happening and consciously intervene to choose a better, healthier alternative. This step was described in my previous article.

The second step, which is far more difficult and challenging, is actually abstaining from highly addictive, artificially created, and calorically concentrated Frankenfoods (to use Dr. Joel Fuhrman's term) which hyperstimulate our brain's pleasure centers. To perform this task requires strategic planning, an understanding of what happens biologically and psychologically when we withdraw from addictive substances, willful determination, and often social and sometimes professional support.

With regards to the first step, strategic planning, you might speculate that the easiest and most painless way of making this transformation is to gradually change your diet over a long period of time, like the gradual transformation of a worm into a butterfly. As it turns out, this is typically not the fastest, easiest, or the most successful way for many people to make the conversion. Have you ever wondered why 12-step programs do not incorporate a gradual withdrawal from addictive substances or stimuli? With good reason—it promotes frequent relapses, extends withdrawal, and delays recovery.

At least some clinical experience has shown that total abstinence, especially when it is accompanied by proper preparation, knowledge of the withdrawal process, and social support, results in higher success rates. Why? Because:

- You avoid the pain of repeated withdrawal cycles,
- You avoid being repeatedly confronted with feelings of self-defeat and decreased self-confidence after relapses,
- You experience the resulting benefits of the conversion more quickly, more powerfully, and more pronounced, and
- You have greater control over cravings for junk foods, which become less intense the longer you abstain.

A "cold-turkey" conversion might seem counterintuitive, but this approach might just offer you your best chance for success. Pushing through withdrawal quickly and experiencing significant benefits on the other side of recovery can help motivate you to "stick to it" for good.

When you only make incremental changes in your diet, you only get tiny improvements to your health and well-being that may not be apparent or detectable by you. For example, you may not notice that adding an apple a day or a spear of broccoli every day does anything to your health and erroneously conclude that it doesn't make any difference. On the other hand, if you make a quick and total conversion to healthy eating, significant, detectable, and often dramatic results occur in the months that follow. For example:

- Symptoms from health issues might diminish or disappear,
- Chronic diseases—such as heart or artery disease—might be slowed, halted, or even reversed,
- Blood pressure and total cholesterol levels might plummet,
- Energy levels might be revitalized,
- Brain fog might dissipate,
- Healthy body weight might be restored, and
- Reliance on medications might be reduced or even eliminated.

These are not trivial or hard-to-detect changes. When you experience these kinds of benefits, you will be strongly motivated to continue. You will also feel rewarded for having made the change.

Of course, you might not be completely successful on your first or subsequent tries at total abstinence. Repeated effort is often required. But don't get discouraged. Most cigarette smokers require a half-dozen to a dozen serious attempts before they quit. We will discuss tips for making an all-out conversion to healthy eating easier in an upcoming article.

Escaping the pleasure trap: Part 3

Another important weapon in your arsenal for escaping the pleasure trap is understanding the addiction and recovery process. You must know what is happening to your body (and brain) during *withdrawal*—the painful period that immediately follows abstinence from an addictive substance. Unless you understand what is happening, when your body screams out and insists that you immediately put an end to the pain and discomfort you are experiencing, you will have little power to resist.

When using an addictive substance for the very first time, the pleasure centers of your brain light up brightly as the dopamine levels in your brain go sky high. (If you are a parent, think back to how your child reacted the very first time you gave him or her ice cream.) However, with repeated use of the addictive substance, the number of dopamine receptors in your brain actually decreases. Your brain develops a "tolerance" for the substance—meaning you don't experience the same "high" as you did in the beginning. This is known as *habituation*.

During habituation, your natural reaction is to try to compensate for a feeling of decreased pleasure by increasing the amount, the frequency of use, and/or the concentration of the addictive substance in an attempt to push pleasure levels up to their previous levels. For example, you eat larger portions of junk food; you eat junk food more often; and/or you select junk food containing higher concentrations of sugar, fat, or salt. This drives addiction. You want to feel that initial rush of pleasure again and again.

When you decide to stop using an addictive substance, you go into withdrawal. During this phase, your feelings of pleasure quickly plummet and descend to levels that are actually far below their pre-use levels. This results in severe mental and physical anguish. You feel miserable.

Because pain and discomfort are built-in biological cues to stop doing what you are doing, your natural instinct is to immediately end abstinence and return to using the offending substance. But your biological cues are misleading you. You are in the midst of the pleasure trap. Your built-in biological instincts for pleasure and pain avoidance are being deceived. They are telling you to stop the pain of withdrawal and return to the pleasure of substance abuse with its resulting self-destructive behavior.

The few days that follow total abstinence are typically the worst and most challenging. Relapses can easily occur. However, if you are persistent—despite any relapses—and eventually push through your withdrawal symptoms, you can then start *recovery*.

During recovery, your feelings of overall happiness and pleasure with life can be healed and be restored to their normal, pre-use levels (unless, of course, the addictive substance was so destructive that it did permanent damage to your brain, your neural circuits, and possibly other parts of your body). Further vigilance is required on your part to guard against "temptation" and relapses.

Here are some suggestions and tips for pushing through withdrawal:

- Recognize that it is normal to feel miserable during the first few days of withdrawal. Discount the voices in your head that are insisting that you quit.
- Remember that withdrawal is of limited duration—perhaps a few weeks in the case of abstinence from junk foods, with the first few days being the worst. "This too will end."
- Get the support of sympathetic family members or friends who can help you keep your resolve during your most challenging moments and safeguard you from relapse.

- Understand that sudden and powerful cravings for junk food will calm down, become less frequent, and become less intense over time.
- Suspend your disbelief that eating a whole-food, plant-based diet cannot possibly be pleasurable (after all, as of yet, you have never really given it a chance).
- Take it on faith that your taste buds will eventually recover so that natural foods will taste good to you.
- Distract your brain by engaging in physical and/or mental activities that keep you mentally and physically occupied during withdrawal.
- Remember that giving in to your cravings will reactivate the addictive pleasure circuits of your brain and reinstate the pleasure trap, thus delaying your progress. As all recovering alcoholics know, you cannot have "just one drink."
- Remember that if you delay going "sober" for too long, the months and years may fly by until you eventually pass through a "one-way door" with irreversible health consequences.
- Recognize that a new, healthy life is only a few weeks away. When you are standing on the side of a mountain, you cannot see the beauty of the amazing panoramic mountain vistas that lie hidden just over the top of the ridge. So, climb on!

This is no trivial battle. Your health and the quality of your life and that of your loved ones hangs in the balance. The stakes are high. Get professional help if you need it to push through withdrawal.

Escaping the pleasure trap: Part 4

Previously, we discussed why your chances of success could be higher if you convert over to healthy eating all at once. However, naively abstaining from all junk food without any prior planning, forethought, or preparation is a plan to fail, not succeed. There are simply too many new skills—such as how to plan for and prepare healthy meals with minimal effort—and too much needed information—such as what food to buy and which recipes you like—to think that you will address pressing hunger pains and urgent cravings by winging it (hunger doesn't wait!). With that in mind, here are a few suggestions that you might find helpful:

- One of the biggest barriers to healthy eating is the fear that you will be deprived of eating foods that taste good to you. Many people "live to eat" instead of "eating to live" and are unwilling to make the "sacrifice" of giving up foods like ice cream, donuts, cake, hamburgers, and fries. To counter this fear, start right away to eat fresh or frozen fruit, including berries, to satisfy your sweet tooth. Then, find vegan or nutritarian recipes you think you might like and try them out. Save the ones you like and create your own recipe collection, no matter how small. With the proper combinations of herbs, spices, and textures, real foods can taste great. Healthy recipes can be found everywhere—in recipe books, such as *The How Not to Die Cookbook* by Dr. Michael Greger, and on websites, such as drfuhrman.com, forksoverknives.com, and engine2diet.com. After you find recipes that you like, prepare them repeatedly until you are confident at making them so you will not be struggling to learn how to cook healthy food when you are under the stress of withdrawal.

- Another barrier to healthy eating is the extra effort people think it will require to eat healthily. Fast food plays on our biological motivation to minimize effort. When we are hungry, nothing is easier than pulling up to the drive-through window of a nearby fast-food restaurant. You don't even have to get out of your car to satisfy your hunger. To address this biological mechanism to minimize effort, make it easy to eat healthy foods by making them readily available at home and by making food planning and preparation super-efficient. Assemble a couple of weeks of menus in advance, create shopping lists, consolidate trips to the grocery store, cook and freeze food in advance, prepare non-cooked items ahead of time and store them in individual containers, double or triple recipes when you cook so you can eat the same food the following day or two without cooking, develop a schedule that distributes the food preparation work load across several days, and enlist the help of your spouse and children in all these tasks.

- Another common misconception about healthy eating is that it is expensive. To address this objection, buy things in bulk from large wholesale clubs or discount stores, like grains and nuts, large bags of pre-washed dark-green lettuces (such as a kale, spinach, and chard mix), fresh or frozen berries, and large bags of frozen vegetables. When you compare how much you are currently spending on meat and dairy products (including milk, yogurt, cheese, ice cream, and eggs), fresh fruit looks very reasonable by comparison. And just one visit to the doctor along with a few lab tests will really make those frozen berries seem inexpensive.

- Change your food environment by getting rid of all junk food and processed food from your house. If tempting but unhealthy food is within arm's reach, you will eat it. Be ruthless. Avoid secretly hiding some of it "just in case." Make it as hard as possible to find and eat junk food. When you are constantly bombarded by junk food temptations, you waste valuable mental and emotional energies having to justify all over again why you are not eating junk food, which risks relapse.

- Accept that the work you do to prepare real food is just a required part of being alive. We only think it is a sacrifice to prepare real food because we are comparing the effort of doing so against the ease of buying and eating unhealthy junk-food. Fast food and junk food is a relatively recent development in the history of mankind. Before the rise of processed foods and hamburger stands in the mid-twentieth century, everyone had to prepare real food three times a day just to feed their families and stay alive. So, don't participate in a pity party. You'll only be doing what human beings have been doing for centuries, but faster and easier with the aid of modern tools and appliances.

- Trust that, after you have been "stone-cold sober" and have refrained from eating junk food for a few weeks, your taste buds will change and your satisfaction in eating real foods will increase. Some studies have even shown that participants rate their gustatory pleasure from eating a whole-food, plant-based diet just as high as when they were eating their previous diet.

- Take the focus of where you get your satisfaction in life off of eating junk food and processed foods. Get your fulfillment from other sources. Explore and develop your talents and interests. Do some service for others. Make your home and the world a better place. Find joy in developing your relationships. Socialize with friends. Do something good so you can feel good. All these things will help you avoid using junk food as an emotional crutch, to break up boredom, or to self-sooth.

- Watch the documentaries and read the books on healthy eating that I have recommended. Not only will they give you the "big picture" regarding *why* you should eat real food, they will arm you with facts, examples, and motivational success stories that will strengthen your resolve. Then go back and watch or read them again and again. Try to absorb every bit of their motivational energy.
- Be sure to have healthy nutritarian snacks readily available in your pantry or refrigerator. These can be things like healthy homemade energy bars, ready-to-eat fruits (such as bananas, apples, pears, peaches, grapes, and fresh and frozen berries), home-made 100 percent whole-wheat bread (individual slices can be kept frozen in the freezer), ready-to-eat raw vegetables, dried fruit (such as raisins and prunes), watermelon and other melons, soy or almond milk, hot-air-popped popcorn (eaten without salt and butter), steel-cut oats with raisins and cinnamon, and raw nuts. A kitchen and pantry devoid of ready-to-eat healthy foods is asking for trouble.
- Outfit your kitchen with the tools and countertop appliances that will make food preparation faster and easier. Purchase or acquire: a set of quality kitchen knives for cutting and chopping vegetables; a dozen small paring knives to cut apples, oranges, and other fruit (so you will always have a clean knife available to cut up some fruit); a small blender for grinding flax and other seeds; a high-speed blender for making fruit smoothies; glass and plastic containers to store the large quantities of food that you prepare in advance; several cutting boards or liners for chopping; small and large colanders (for washing fruits, berries, and vegetables); specialty tools like garlic presses and mango cutters; a heavy duty bread maker and a wheat mill for making whole-wheat bread and rolls from raw wheat kernels; a large pot for making a week's worth of soup; automatic pressure cookers for cooking grains, beans, vegetables, and other food; and even a second refrigerator and a deep freeze so you will have room to store all the things you buy and prepare (modern refrigerators and freezers use very little electricity).

- Find other sympathetic souls who can teach you how to eat healthily and who can give you support and encouragement. Lean on them heavily, especially during withdrawal and recovery.

By following these suggestions, you will be better prepared to achieve success when you finally "flip the switch" to a completely healthy way of eating.

What you leave behind when you stop eating junk food

Many people are reluctant to change what they eat because it requires they stop eating "foods" that give them pleasure but are harmful to their bodies—namely, hamburgers, French fries, candies, ice cream, cakes, donuts, cookies, crackers, white bread, white rice, foods with added oils and fats, and many other highly processed foods. They also do not want to give up meat, dairy (including milk, ice cream, cheese, and yogurt), and eggs, even though all these things are strongly associated with cancer, high blood pressure, heart disease, type-2 diabetes, and other illnesses. Many people are addicted to junk foods and don't even know it.

But aside from a few short moments of temporary pleasure—which is *all* that junk food has to offer—what are you really leaving behind when you stop eating junk food? You leave behind:

- Nutritionally bankrupt foods that supply your body with *macronutrients* (protein, carbohydrates, and/or fat) but few or no *micronutrients*, elements which are essential to good health and disease prevention.
- Foods with high amounts of added salt.
- Foods that almost always have added sugar in them. Excess sugar is converted into fat and over time can lead to type 2 diabetes and an increased risk of cancer.
- Foods containing added preservatives, processing agents, emulsifiers, enhancers, food colorings, and other chemicals that your body does not recognize that are suspected of causing harm to your health.

- Foods that leave you feeling empty or wanting more, especially just a couple of hours later when their refined carbohydrates have been digested and you feel a "sugar low."
- Foods that cause constipation and other digestive problems, due to their lack of fiber.
- Foods that feed the wrong kind of gut bacteria in your intestines, leading to a compromised immune system and other problems.
- A bigger waistline. If you eat junk foods, you are almost guaranteed to become overweight and experience the health issues associated with obesity. One reason for this is because junk food is addictive, and you can never eat enough junk food to satisfy your addictions. Another reason is because junk food contains high levels of fat, sugar, and other refined carbohydrates, which are quickly stored as fat in your body.
- Foods containing processed oils and fats that are made up of mostly omega-6 fatty acids, which skews the critical ratio of omega-6 fatty acids to omega-3 fatty acids in your diet. These fats are also quickly absorbed and stored in your body as fat.
- A sudden flood of oxidative stress to your cells, which wreaks havoc on the cellular level because there are few or no phytonutrients and antioxidants to neutralize them.
- The suffering, pain, financial costs, loss of freedom, and depression that come when you contract a serious preventable disease or illness.
- A shorter lifespan. Research shows that those who eat the standard American diet live shorter lives than those who eat a whole-food, plant-based diet.

So, as you can see, you've left nothing of real value behind when you give up junk food.

Is healthy eating extreme?

Eating healthily may be out of sync with how most Americans eat today, and some may even say that eating such a diet is extreme. But let's look at the facts.

Consider the top two killers of Americans today: heart disease (633,842 deaths a year) and cancer (595,930 deaths a year). The first symptom of heart disease for many people is a heart attack. Many of those heart attacks are immediately fatal. If you do survive, you may require a stint or bypass operation.

With a bypass, the surgeon makes a long incision down your chest along your breastbone, cracks open your rib cage to expose the heart, and temporarily stops your heart while you are put on a heart-lung machine. The surgeon then takes a healthy section of a blood vessel (often by cutting open and removing a blood vessel from your leg), and attaches the ends of it above and below the blocked artery in your heart so blood flows around it.

This is a major operation. You will likely spend a couple of days in intensive care and several more days in the hospital. You will have a breathing tube in your throat until you can breathe on your own. If all goes well, you might be discharged from the hospital in a week, although you may find it difficult to perform your usual daily tasks for some time.

Besides expiring on the operating table during the procedure, the risks of this operation include, among others, infections of the wound, irregular heart rhythm, bleeding, stroke, kidney problems, and additional heart attacks if a clot is broken loose during surgery.

Did you know that leading cardiologists have said that heart disease is a largely preventable disease if we just changed our diet and got adequate exercise?

Now consider the second leading killer of Americans today: cancer. Those who have had to fight cancer know the extremes to which they are called to endure with chemotherapy (strong poisons that kill not only your cancer cells, but your immune system cells as well) and radiation treatment. Many who have been through these treatments swear they will never go through them again.

And then there are the operations to remove the cancerous tumors or organs of your body, leaving you scarred, maimed, and without those critical organs, causing debilitations and limitations you must live with for the rest of your life. Amazingly, cancer used to be a relatively rare disease, but in modern times, it has blossomed into the second leading cause of death.

Many nutritionists and researchers are convinced that eating a healthy plant-based diet can prevent many cancers because it provides your body with antioxidants, phytonutrients, and other substances which fight and kill cancer cells before they can multiply into deadly tumors or spread throughout your body.

Moreover, surgical and pharmacological treatments for heart disease and cancer do not guarantee that the diseases will never come back. That is because they don't address the *cause* of the disease. All they do is treat the *symptoms*. The reasons why the cancer or heart disease appeared in the first place are *not* addressed. Recurrence is therefore common.

So, you tell me what is more extreme? Eating a natural, whole-food, plant-based diet, or having a lethal heart attack—leaving your spouse and children broken-hearted and perhaps financially destitute—having a bypass operation or some other invasive medical procedure, or having cancer treatments that some say are worse to endure then the cancer?

WEEK 4

"You're a real fighter. Keep up the good work!"

About the "Aligning the stars in your favor" series

The articles in the next two weeks are designed to help align the stars in your favor by making certain changes in your life. These changes, when joined together, generate concentrated power that will help you choose to eat more healthily.

Aligning the stars in your favor: Controlling your food environment

You may not be able to control the larger social and cultural environment that you are immersed in, but you can change the environment where you spend most of your time—your home. If you are serious about changing over to healthy eating, you should purge your house of all unhealthy foods and replace them with healthy foods. This means going through your refrigerator, freezer, and pantry and getting rid of:

- All junk food,
- All processed foods, including most packaged and processed foods; packaged breakfast cereals; foods with added sugar, fat, or salt; and foods stripped of their fiber (juice, for example, has no fiber),
- All foods with highly processed carbs, such as white bread, white rice, white potatoes, cake and brownie mixes, white flour, and sugar,
- Cooking oils, including olive oil (these are 100 percent fat and have little significant nutritional value), and
- All animal products, including meat, dairy (including milk, ice cream, yogurt, and cheese), and eggs.

Why? Because if unhealthy food is staring you in the face, you will be more likely to eat it. You shouldn't have tempting, unhealthy foods inside your home. Instead, make it easy to reach for healthy foods.

Replace unhealthy foods with their healthy counterparts. This means stocking up on:

- Whole grains, such as quinoa, steel cut oats, brown rice, whole-wheat pasta, corn (fresh or frozen), whole-wheat tortillas (for bean burritos and wraps), whole-wheat buns (for vegan burgers), popcorn (for the hot-air popper, not bagged microwave popcorn), and whole-wheat bread,
- A plant-based milk substitute, such as soy milk or almond milk,
- Fresh or frozen berries, such as strawberries, blueberries, raspberries, and blackberries,
- Other fruit, fresh or frozen, such as apples, oranges, tangerines, pears, bananas, grapes, peaches, cantaloupe, watermelon, plums, pineapple, avocados, cherries, apricots, kiwifruit, dates, cranberries, lemons, limes, and pomegranates,
- Fresh and frozen vegetables, including a variety of dark leafy greens, broccoli, tomatoes, carrots, peppers (red, green, yellow, or orange), peas (fresh snap or frozen), asparagus, green beans (fresh or frozen), Brussels sprouts, fresh mushrooms (which should be cooked before eating), celery, radishes, parsley, red and yellow onions, purple cabbage, green cabbage, scallions (green onions), cauliflower, sweet potatoes, cucumbers, and garlic,
- Dried fruits, such as raisins and prunes,
- Raw, unsalted, unroasted nuts, including almonds, walnuts, pistachios, cashews, pecans, sunflower seeds, pumpkin seeds, chia seeds, flax seeds, and sesame seeds,
- Almond butter or all-natural peanut butter (refrigerate after opening to help prevent the oils in them from going rancid),
- Spices and other cooking ingredients, including tomato paste, canned tomatoes, and nutritional yeast, and
- Beans and other lentils (canned, if you don't want to bother with cooking them yourself, if they are low in salt), including back beans, kidney beans, pinto beans, garbanzo beans (chickpeas), white beans, and other legumes called for by your healthy recipes.

If this transition is too big to make all at once, do it piecemeal. But refrain from restocking unhealthy foods. This last step is just as important as your initial "house cleaning." If you return and buy ice cream at the store, for example, you might as well consider it eaten before you reach the checkout counter.

Align the stars in your favor by ridding your house of nutrient-deficient foods and controlling your environment.

Aligning the stars in your favor: The power of routines

An episode entitled "Future Shock" of the old TV sitcom *Home Improvement* poked fun at the routines Tim followed every day and portrayed some funny consequences that might occur if he broke those routines. Aside from Tim's personal routines, all businesses run on procedures or routines that are repeated daily, weekly, or on some other schedule. They provide the necessary activities for the business to function. Although you might think that having a set of routines that you follow in your personal life will make your life too rigid and stymie your creativity, spontaneity, or freedom, I have found just the opposite to be the case—it knocks out the necessary grunt work in life so that I *can* be creative and spontaneous in the remaining time I have every day, which is maximized due to the efficiencies of the routines.

Harness the power of routines to do food preparation, shopping, and meal planning. For example, prepare a week's worth of healthy soups, veggies, nuts, and fruit on the weekend and store them in individual containers that you can simply take out and eat at mealtimes. This will help assure that you and your family eat healthily every day. When you are starving at meal times is not a good time to decide if you will send out for pizza or spend thirty minutes preparing a healthy meal. Prepare your meals as much as possible ahead of time to minimize the time that it takes to put food on your table.

As you execute your routines repeatedly, you will become more proficient at them. They will eventually become automatic, which means they are more likely to be performed, and the tasks themselves will not seem as difficult or intimidating as they once did. For example, the first time I prepared vegetable-bean soup from a recipe, it took me two or three hours and was pretty intimidating. Now, I can whip up a week's worth in my sleep.

You gain a new appreciation for just how much routines contribute to your life when they are disrupted, such as when a family member comes to visit for a few days or when you fall ill and cannot perform them.

Align the stars in your favor by establishing nutritional routines for healthy eating.

Aligning the stars in your favor: Making deposits into your Personal Health Account (PHA)

No, not the Health Savings Account (HSA) account that is associated with your health insurance plan, but the health account your body maintains based on how well you care for it. You make *deposits* into the latter account when you eat something healthy, get daily exercise, go to bed early, manage stress, avoid smoking, and wear disposable gloves when you fill your lawn mower with gasoline, use household cleaners, or handle other chemicals. You make *withdrawals* from that account when you eat junk food, live a sedentary lifestyle, get too little sleep, fail to manage stress, smoke, and handle carcinogens with your bare hands. Just like with real savings accounts, an occasional withdrawal will not change your overall financial standing, but persistent, repeated withdrawals with few or no deposits will.

For example, you make a deposit into your PHA every time you eat beans. Eating just a cup of beans, chickpeas, or lentils every day for three months can slow a person's resting heart rate as much as spending 250 hours on a treadmill and is probably the most important dietary predictor of survival in older persons around the world—an 8 percent decrease in premature death risk for each daily ounce intake. One thing that Blue Zones (areas around the world with the greatest longevity) have in common is their residents regularly eat legumes (beans, lentils, peas, and chickpeas).

You also make deposits into your PHA when you eat fruit or vegetables. A seven-year study of more than half a million Chinese adults found that those who ate fruit regularly cut their risk from dying from cardiovascular disease by roughly one-third. If half of Americans ate a single more serving of fruits and vegetables a day, 20,000 less people would die from cancer. Imagine that—making just one more deposit a day into their PHA could save the lives of 20,000 people a year in America alone. That's almost seven times the number of people who died from the September 11, 2001 terrorist attack who would be saved every year!

Men make withdrawals from their PHAs every time they eat dairy foods, such as milk, yogurt, cheese, or ice cream. Dairy increases a man's risk of getting prostate cancer by about a third. And for women who have had breast cancer, just one serving of dairy a day can increase their chance of dying from the disease by 49 percent.

What happens when you bankrupt your Personal Health Account and run up huge deficits? The answer, of course, is poor health. As Dr. Joel Fuhrman likes to say, "Good health cannot be bought—it must be earned through healthy eating." If you run your car into the ground, you don't know just how much longer it will last before it breaks down, but eventually it will, and most likely, much sooner than it otherwise would. On the other hand, maintaining your car and fueling it with pure, clean, unadulterated gasoline will greatly increase its lifespan and reliability.

So every time you pick up a fork, lift up a slice of pizza, or dip into a carton of ice cream, ask yourself, "Am I making a deposit into my Personal Health Account, or am I making a withdrawal?" Then, periodically ask yourself, "What is the status of *my* Personal Health Account?"

Aligning the stars in your favor: Combating emotional eating

According to the Mayo Clinic, emotional eating is "eating as a way to suppress or soothe negative emotions, such as stress, anger, fear, boredom, sadness, and loneliness" (see the article, "Weight loss: Gain control of emotional eating" on mayoclinic.org). We eat because of the way it makes us *feel*, not because we are hungry. Emotional eating can easily become an emotional crutch—an easy way to counteract uncomfortable emotions.

While everyone does emotional eating at one time or another, your emotions can become so tied to your eating habits that you automatically reach for a treat whenever you're angry or stressed without even thinking about what you're doing. This, of course, leads to unwanted weight gain.

One way to combat negative emotions, such as stress, anger, fear, boredom, sadness, and loneliness, is to do something for others. "When we *do* good, we *feel* good." Feeling good about ourselves chases away those negative emotions. Doing something good for others forces us to interact with them, helps us to feel useful and wanted, strengthens our positive view of ourselves, and makes us less susceptible to emotional eating.

This is not a sermon, but practical advice. Take your kids to the park, help your spouse with the housework, befriend a neighbor, give an extra generous tip to a server, express your love and appreciation to a family member, lift someone who is feeling down, and smile more. What you do *during* the day will help determine how you will feel at the *end* of the day. Being tired from helping others feels different than being tired for other reasons.

Aligning the stars in your favor: Making swift course corrections

Being human, we're not always going to eat perfectly healthy all the time. Instead of striving for perfection, which, as I mentioned previously, is often unproductive, we should strive for progress and greater consistency in healthy eating. But sometimes life's circumstances and other events such as binge eating or emotional eating combine to send us into a spiral of unhealthy or excessive eating. When this happens, rather than bemoaning our self-control, becoming discouraged, and giving up hope, make a quick course correction. The next day, start eating healthily again, get more sleep at night, exercise, and rid your house of the tempting snacks and food that steered you wrong. Quickly getting back on course is a skill that all those who pursue healthy living need to acquire.

Your bathroom scale can help keep you honest in recognizing when you have potentially veered off course. After you have overeaten or gone on a binge, you already know that you have veered off course, but sometimes you just want to sweep it under the rug and pretend it didn't happen. Self-denial just makes it that much easier to overeat or go on a binge the next day. By stepping on the scale, you are given a reality check and a signal that you need to make an immediate course correction.

Guiding yourself back on course without berating yourself when you take a wrong turn is the compassionate way of encouraging yourself to make progress toward your goal of healthy eating.

Aligning the stars in your favor: Taming your sweet tooth

I received a postcard in my mailbox the other day advertising an event sponsored by a dentist for an upcoming presentation on a dental procedure. The ad prominently mentioned that "We will satisfy your sweet tooth" with donuts, ice cream, and the other treats. That got me thinking. Can a sweet tooth ever be satisfied? I have had a so-called "sweet tooth" my entire life. I've always loved desserts, cookies, sweets, and treats.

The problem is, sugar is addictive, and when combined with fat, it is even more addictive. As with all addictions, you can never completely satisfy or remove the addition by giving in to it. When you do this, the cravings come back as strong as before. I'm not sure if there is a Twelve Step program for recovering sugar addicts, but one thing is sure: indulging your sweet tooth "just this once," like a person who wants "just one drink" who has been living sober, does not work. It triggers your brain's addiction mechanisms all over again and quickly leads to more indulgence.

While eliminating all foods with added sugar is hard, it is easier than constantly teasing yourself with "occasional" treats—after all, how often is occasional? Those indulgences make it that much harder the next day to avoid them, and they rekindle the fires of former addictions. The sugar high and sugar low are known bodily chemical reactions to eating sugar. When you reach that low, you want to eat more sugar.

Eating a nutritarian diet consisting of whole grains, beans and other legumes, fruits, vegetables, nuts, and seeds, and avoiding meat, dairy, eggs, highly processed foods, and junk food, stabilizes swings in your blood sugar level. You don't experience the extreme highs and lows that plague sugar eaters. You may also discover that you have greater endurance.

After you have been eating healthily for a few weeks, foods with natural sugar in them, such as fruits and even some vegetables, begin to taste very sweet. You can sweeten up your morning oatmeal, for example, by adding a few raisins instead of a spoonful of brown sugar. Naturally sweet whole foods come packaged with a lot of fiber, so they are absorbed more slowly into your bloodstream.

If you have an intense craving for sweets, reach for fruits and berries—nature's sweets—or make yourself some "Fudgy No-bake Brownies" made from dates, almond butter, ground walnuts, and cocoa powder (see the recipe in Dr. Greger's, *The How Not to Die Cookbook*).

Aligning the stars in your favor: Avoiding wandering eyes in the grocery store

According to some studies, grocery stores are typically filled 70 percent or more with highly processed foods. For example, most of today's grocery stores have a whole aisle devoted to chips, another devoted to candies, another to ice cream and desserts, and another to breakfast cereals. Aside from aisles filled with junk foods, other aisles are filled with highly refined convenience foods that are stripped of fiber and micronutrients and have added sugar, fat, and salt. These "foods" are packaged in colorful, highly enticing containers that promise short preparation times and amazing culinary pleasure. So, what's a brain to do that is exposed to all this?

Marketers know how your brain will respond—put it in your cart—and Americans do by the cartload! What you need is a strategy to minimize the impulse to buy these products. One effective strategy is to control where your eyes fall in the grocery store. Marketers pay more to have their products placed at eye level on grocery store shelves because they know that if you look at their products, you will see the marketing hype on their packages and be influenced to buy their products.

In Greek mythology, the Sirens were dangerous creatures, who lured nearby sailors with their enchanting music and singing voices to shipwreck on the rocky coast of their island (Wikipedia). Don't let the singing Sirens of the processed food industry's alluring food packages cause a shipwreck of poor health in your voyage through life.

The next time you go to the grocery store, arm yourself with a shopping list of the healthy items you want to buy. Keep your eyes in the middle of the aisle and pick up your pace as you rush to get to the fresh produce section at the back of the store. Avoid going by the bakery and drooling over and smelling the fresh donuts or passing by the freezers filled with ice cream. Talk to yourself as these products call out to you and tell yourself that you eat only healthy, real foods grown by Mother Nature. These suggestions may seem facetious, but they all have a kernel of truth in them. You only buy the things that you see. So, stop seeing what you shouldn't be buying!

WEEK 5

"Can you believe it? A month already. You're well underway"

Aligning the stars in your favor: Changing your concept of "What is food?"

While I was washing the kale, collard greens, Swiss chard, and parsley from my garden the other day, I suddenly realized that I actually considered what I was washing to be food. A few years ago, I would have looked at a pile of greens like that and thought "rabbit food" or "salad greens that have no taste and don't really satisfy." I was entirely ignorant that dark green leafy vegetables are some of the healthiest and most nutrient-dense foods on the planet.

That same day, while I was in the checkout line at a local fresh-produce store, a couple behind me noticed what I was buying (some dry beans and tons of fruits and vegetables) and asked me if I was vegan. I said that I was (well, I am actually a nutritarian, but I didn't feel like explaining the difference at the time), and they became very excited that they had encountered a like-minded person. I saw what they were buying and said "You definitely know how to eat healthily yourselves!"

But how would the typical American view a grocery store checkout conveyor belt filled with dry beans, whole grains, fruits, nuts, seeds, and vegetables? I sometimes imagine what they are thinking when I am checking out at the store: "You eat only that? Where is the meat? Where is the white bread and other bakery items? Where are the packages of processed foods? Where is the milk, cheese, and ice cream? Where are the deli meats? Where are the breakfast cereals? Where are the crackers, cookies, and snacks? WHAT ARE YOU GOING TO EAT?"

Yes, my concept of "what is food?" has changed over the last couple of years. I now view highly processed foods, fast foods, and junk foods as fake food, nutrient-deficient food, or artificial food that are masquerading as food. I now see meat, dairy, and eggs as animal products that come with a very high price tag from a health, humanitarian, and environmental point of view. I now look at packaged breakfast cereals and think "why would I eat that sugared-up, machine-generated fluff when I can eat real, whole-grain breakfast cereals, like steel-cut oats with raisons and cinnamon?" While fake food sometimes still calls out to me, I combat the urge to eat it with the knowledge of what eating real food will do for me.

Aligning the stars in your favor: Choosing to like healthy foods

It amazes me to see how food preferences differ across cultures and even within our own country. Chinese food differs from Indian food. German food differs from English food. Polish food differs from Vietnamese food.

If you are a Southerner, you love grits, succotash, chicken fried steak with white gravy, and fried green tomatoes. If you are a Texan, you love pulled barbeque pork, big steaks, big plates of Tex-Mex, and large bowls of Texas chili.

What is one person's disgusting food is another's delicacy. Most westerners love cheese, but many Chinese hate it; however, in China, sea cucumber is an expensive delicacy. I love the taste of root beer, but in Argentina, people think it tastes like bad medicine. On the other hand, they love tripe, which is cooked cow stomach.

Scientists believe our tongues can sense five basic tastes: sweet, sour, bitter, salty, and umami (which means "pleasant savory taste" in Japanese). So, if we all come equipped with the same standard tasting equipment on the surface of our tongues, what accounts for the huge disparities in the foods people like and dislike?

To answer that, I believe we must look at the foods we ate growing up and were taught to like. What parent has not tried to get their infant to like a new jar of baby food by taking a bite and saying "mmm" or "yummy"? My grandkids love freshly milled whole-wheat pancakes with homemade syrup because that is what I fed them most Sundays for lunch after church when they were growing up. But recently when I tried to expand their repertoire of healthy foods—of which syrup was not a member—the younger ones acted like I was serving up Chinese sea cucumbers. Why? Their brains had been trained to like certain foods over a period of years, and they did not want to deviate from the foods to which they were accustomed. They "knew" what they liked and disliked.

We are hardwired to like sweet tasting foods, probably because they are concentrated sources of energy, and to dislike bitter-tasting foods, which may indicate spoilage. But we can consciously override our innate distaste for bitter foods and learn to like things like sauerkraut and cocoa. We learn our food preferences from our culture and from the family in which we grew up. Taste preferences reside in our *brains*, not in our *mouths*.

If that is true, can we learn to reprogram our taste preferences? I believe we can.

To do so, though, involves consciously overriding our thought processes while we repeatedly expose ourselves to the new foods over a period of time. For example, each time we eat the new food, we should try to sense all the different tastes and flavors while telling our brain, "This is different, but I like it!" Not all foods have to taste sweet or caress our tongues like ice cream. You can learn to enjoy eating wholesome foods such as intact grains, beans, fruits, vegetables, raw nuts, and seeds. A few years ago, I only ate corn on the cob after slathering it with lots of butter. Today, I love eating corn on the cob with no butter on it at all—it tastes quite sweet and provides a satisfying variety of flavors and textures.

To put your brain on the fast track for liking healthy foods, eat them exclusively for a couple of months. Your "taste buds" will readjust and you will start to sense and enjoy the tastes of real foods.

Aligning the stars in your favor: Building emotional and social support structures

To make a life-altering change to healthy eating requires more than just a heartfelt desire. The temptation to eat junk food can be found on every corner, in every office building, and in every place of business (candy bars are even sold at the checkout line at cloth stores). Powerful cultural and social norms about what is "normal" and "good" to eat must be confronted at every social and family occasion where food is served. You may ask, "How can I eat this way when everyone else is eating differently? Won't I be seen as strange, or worse, as having gone off the deep end?"

Tactically, this is where a little finesse can help. Be preemptive. Announce to your friends and family that you are trying to eat healthier. You don't have to use emotionally charged words like "vegetarian" or "vegan" or unknown words like "nutritarian." Just tell them that you are trying to eat healthier and that research shows that eating more fruits, vegetables, whole grains, beans, nuts, and seeds brings better health and staves off disease. If questioned further, refer them to a couple of great websites where they can go to learn more: nutritionfacts.org and drfuhrman.com. When offered dessert, you don't have to go into a diatribe on why sugar is bad. Simply say, "No thanks. I'm watching my sugar intake [or calories] right now." Many of them will secretly admire your self-control.

Besides polite but honest explanations given to others in social situations, there is still more you can do to build up social support to eat healthily. Ask your spouse if he/she will support you in your efforts to eat healthier, even if he/she is not ready to make a change in that direction right now. If your spouse is unwilling, ask a trusted friend. What you want is someone who will lend you social and emotional support, encouragement, and praise as you make progress and reach small milestones, whatever those may be.

When we know our behavior is being monitored, we are more likely to change our behavior—we have a degree of personal accountability to another person who is important to us. If we binge in social isolation, who is going to know or care? When we know that we are not taking on the world alone, that we have a cheerleader who will praise our honest efforts, celebrate milestones, and help us get back up on the horse after we fall, we are more likely to continue.

A recent *LinkedIn* article discussed an ingenious new model of health care that was started by a Harvard Medical School student. Among other things, that new model incorporates the concept of a Health Coach—a friend and a cheerleader who proactively managed each patient's health, even doing things like taking diabetic patients to the grocery store to help them shop for the right foods, running Zumba classes, and conducting smoking-cessation clinics. In other words, Health Coaches provided a strong social and emotional support structure. The outcomes of this model were successful on all measures.

Try to find someone who will be your own personal Health Coach.

Aligning the stars in your favor: Avoiding one-way doors

If you want to have continuous health in your life, you must avoid going through one-way doors. A one-way door is any preventable disease that permanently alters the quality of your life. For example, if you get cancer and must have a vital organ surgically removed, then you have gone through a one-way door. Or if you get Type 2 diabetes and lose your vision or have a foot amputated, you have gone through a one-way door. Your life is permanently changed and your ability to do things you previously did is reduced or cut off. There is no going back after the fact.

How can you peer into the future to avoid going through one-way doors? You can't. What you can do is set yourself on a path in life that ensures you will by-pass any *preventable* one-way doors. This requires a measure of wisdom on your part to identify what that path is and then the courage to walk down it. The trick is to make the change before it is too late—before you actually go through your first one-way door, or before you set things in motion that guarantee that you will go through a one-way door. Because you don't know how near in your future that door may be, you are better off taking action now to set yourself on that path.

Unfortunately, young people have many things that work against them in seeing the need to do this:

- They are typically blessed with good health right out of the box in life, so they take their health *for granted*, thinking it is the normal state of affairs that will continue forever without any effort on their part.
- They don't have the *hindsight* of having lived several decades of life. They think that disease and health problems are a long way off, if they ever come at all, so why worry. They never have suffered through serious illness or disease, so they don't understand how vulnerable they really are.
- They are *preoccupied* with the pressing affairs of life, such as work, school, family, social life, and entertainment. They feel they have more important things to concern themselves with.
- They believe that *luck is on their side* and that the odds are in their favor. "I'm healthy now. Look at this physique! I feel great! I don't believe that I will be one of those unfortunate people who will be struck down later."
- They do not comprehend just how *life-altering* a serious illness can be. They have little experience with the pain, suffering, time, financial expense, anxiety, loss of livelihood, loss of physical freedom, and the constriction in overall enjoyment in life that serious illness brings. After all, how many young people today can list all the *serious* consequences of diabetes? They encounter healthy looking diabetics every day, so what's the big deal?
- They *naively believe* that modern medicine can reverse all but the most fatal prognoses. "If you get diabetes, medicine has an

answer for you. All you have to do is follow it, and you will be alright."

What the young have working in their favor are their young, healthy bodies. Young bodies, like new cars, can often take a beating from dietary abuse for years before breaking down and blowing a valve or losing an axle. Bodies are amazing creations with incredible resilience and powers of restoration. This resiliency gives teens and young adults a brief window of opportunity to learn why *they*—not their parents, society, the food industry, or the government—are responsible for their health and to learn that the food they eat and don't eat has serious consequences for today and tomorrow.

Before I went through one of those one-way doors with my cancer operations, I naively believed that the surgeon's predicted lifelong limitations and handicaps simply would not happen to me. After all, I was otherwise strong, active, and healthy. I also didn't believe that I would be bedridden for several days and away from my job for the first five to six weeks after leaving the hospital. I guess I had seen too many movies in which the hero is shot and stands right back up and keeps on going. But the consequences of the surgery came just as the surgeon had predicted. It was a humbling experience. I now fear and respect those one-way doors much more keenly than I used to.

In fact, I want to slam shut any future one-way doors that otherwise might await me by eating the healthiest foods on the planet. I only wish that I had known what I now know many decades earlier. Hopefully, those years of ignorance did not set in motion additional permanent damage to my health. Only time will tell.

Take action now to keep your future avoidable one-way doors tightly shut in your life!

Aligning the stars in your favor: Treating your body with respect

Our bodies are miraculous machines. There are over 37.2 trillion cells in our bodies. The average human brain has 100 billion neurons, which is half the number of estimated stars in the Milky Way. We have 100,000 miles of blood vessels in our bodies, which is almost half the distance to the moon. Our heart beats 80 times per minute, which is over 42 million times a year. Every day, we pump 440 gallons of blood through each of our kidneys. Our lung contains 700 million alveoli. A square inch of our skin has 1,300 nerve cells. Each of our eyes has 110 to 130 million receptors to perceive light. The amazing list goes on and on.

But how has our culture taught us to treat our bodies? Does it teach us to respect our bodies, or does it promote pushing the pedal to the metal by using our bodies to pursue pleasure without regard to consequences? What do fast food advertisements, for example, promote? It's not just food—it's pleasure. But one wonders at what cost? And how does our throw-away culture carry over into the way we treat our bodies? Do we nutritionally abuse out bodies like some people run their cars into the ground?

A commitment to healthy eating is based on having a deep respect for our bodies. This means knowing and appreciating the amazing machines that Mother Nature has endowed us with, understanding the sound principles of nutrition on which our health depends, and being disciplined to eat healthy foods and avoid things that are harmful to bodies. Respecting our bodies doesn't mean the exclusion of all pleasure in life, but it does exclude the mentality of reckless abandonment of everything in the quest to seek maximum physical pleasure at the expense of our bodies.

Aligning the stars in your favor: Avoiding the need for medical care

When you walk into a hospital or doctor's office, the first thing they want to see is your money. Even with employer-sponsored health insurance, employees often pay significant premiums every month for their health insurance, whether they use their plan or not, and when they do, they pay high deductibles and percentages.

Doctors are busy. A recent national news article reported that, on average, doctors interrupt patients and stop listening after only 11 seconds. In a recent survey of 1000 physicians, six out of ten agreed with the statement, "My visits with patients are often too short for me to answer their questions and treat them effectively." Doctors are pressured to keep visits short so they can maximize the number of patients they see in a day. In fact, 13 to 16 minutes is the most reported length of time doctors spend with patients.

A major news network reported on a recent study conducted by Johns Hopkins that showed that more than 250,000 people in the United States die every year because of medical mistakes. This made it the third leading cause of death after heart disease and cancer. Let's see. That's 83 times the number of people who died in the September 11, 2001 attacks on America! If we had 83 terrorist attacks a year on U.S. soil like the September 11th attacks, would we be concerned?

Besides medical mistakes, as reported by a leading consumer magazine, every year an estimated 648,000 people in the U.S. develop infections during their stay in the hospital. The Centers for Disease Control and Prevention (CDC) also reports that about 75,000 people a year die from those mistakes.

Is your jaw starting to drop yet?

Based on these facts alone, would you rather stay healthy, stay home, and keep more of your Ben Franklins, or would you rather open your wallet and take your chances to become one of those people who are made sick or killed by the medical profession? I'd rather take good care of my body so I seldom need medical care in the first place.

Aligning the stars in your favor: Getting over your fear of eating fruits

Some people are afraid of eating very much raw fruit because they believe they will gain weight from the sugar it contains. So they dabble with eating a tiny amount, treating it as if it were a calorie-laden double-fudge sundae. Some of these same individuals then turn around and consume foods like yogurt, meat, cheese, salad dressings, mayonnaise, luncheon meats, chocolate chip cookies, ice cream, tortilla chips, and milk, all of which have a lot of fat in them (not to mention sugar). Fat has more than twice as many calories per gram as carbohydrates and proteins—9 calories compared to 4 calories. If anything ought to be scrutinized from a calorie point of view, it is foods that are high in fat (especially animal products, which are high in saturated fat) and processed foods that are high in refined carbs and added sugars that are quickly converted into body fat.

While it may be possible to eat too many calories by loading up on fruit, you will unlikely have this problem. Nature packages the sugar in fruit with lots of fiber and other valuable nutrients. Because fiber is bulky, it fills up your stomach, giving you a full sensation, and it seems to bind up some of the calories with it that are then flushed down the toilet. Fiber also causes the sugar in the fruit to be released more slowly into your bloodstream so your liver doesn't have to trigger excess hormones to convert the sugar into fat.

Eating fruit crowds out the eating of other foods, just due to the limited capacity of your stomach. Sure, if you gorge on fruit and then round out the rest of your meal with high-fat foods, junk foods, and highly processed foods, you will gain weight. But simply eating more fruit may actually lead to weight loss because you have less room for unhealthy, calorically dense foods.

I eat a lot of strawberries, blackberries, and tomatoes (which are considered fruits by scientists) from my garden in the summertime, along with large slices of watermelon from the store, with little effect on my overall weight. I also eat a variety of other fruits from the produce section of the market every day as part of my diet.

Of course, when you first increase your intake of fruit, you might see your weight increase a pound or two on your bathroom scale just from the weight of all the fiber that you have eaten that is in transit, but this is not a permanent part of your body mass.

So, get over your fear of eating fruit. Instead, instill a fear of eating junk foods that *will* cause weight gain when they are eaten without a second thought. Fruit has so many benefits to your health that you should eat a *variety* of it every day in your diet. Cheers to Mother Nature's best!

WEEK 6

"You've shown you're serious about this.
Keep it up!"

Are you on track for a serious train wreck?

Suppose you are traveling on a cross-country train and the conductor suddenly announces that it is on a collision course with another train coming from the opposite direction on the same track. Would you interrupt what you were doing, evaluate your options, and take action, or would you pretend that everything is fine, deny the reality, and return to your dining car to continue eating your morning brunch? Is the latter what we do when we deny that the dietary course we are on will lead to serious health disasters down the road?

For many years, I did just that—ate the standard American diet (SAD) and pretended that everything was just fine—not so much out of denial but out of ignorance. I consumed junk foods, fast foods, and processed foods as a major part of my diet. I was happily streaking across the countryside in my cozy train cabin, feeling safe and secure, not realizing that I was headed for a serious train wreck.

One day that train wreck came. I was diagnosed with two different forms of deadly cancer in the organs of my body within a two week period. My life was suddenly shattered, and my former priorities were scattered around the wreckage like shredded household furniture in the aftermath of a tornado. I faced a whole new reality—one that directly threatened my life. Only then did I start to take my diet more seriously and begin an intense study of healthy eating.

Do not wait until you experience a train wreck in your life before you learn about healthy eating and change how you eat. Stop denying that your diet has everything to do with your health, your vitality, your longevity, and your chances of incurring many serious and debilitating diseases. Take action now to cross over to a track that is free and clear for the rest of your life—before it is too late.

We are not carnivorous apes

Our closest living relative in the animal kingdom—chimpanzees (not apes!)—eat mostly fruits and leaves (a plant-based diet). They get very little of their diet from eating insects, bark, eggs, nuts, and the flesh of other small animals. While technically speaking chimpanzees are omnivores because they sometimes eat non-plant foods, if you classify animals based on what they mostly eat, chimps are frugivores.

A comparison of frugivores and omnivores uncovers many distinct differences, such as: omnivore teeth and jaws are very different from frugivore teeth and jaws; omnivores have much stronger stomach acid; omnivores have front "hands" that are hoofs, claws, or paws while frugivores have hands with fingers that are perfect for picking and peeling fruits and plants; and omnivores have intestines that are about nine times smaller in length to prevent meat from putrefying in their gut if it isn't moved through quickly.

But what about our so-called "canine" teeth? Close inspection shows that these teeth are rounded and are utterly useless for ripping flesh and meat.

Anatomically, we fit all the requirements of a frugivore, not an omnivore. If we were a true omnivore, we would have to change our appearance and physiology.

So, don't be taken in by the argument that we were designed to be meat-eaters. Anatomically, we were designed to be plant-eaters.

What's wrong with my mirror?

The national news recently reported on a British study of men and women's body image in which 60 percent of the men and 30 percent of the women who were overweight or obese did not see themselves as overweight or obese.

A couple of weeks ago, I went shopping for men's T-shirts. I had to buy "small" size shirts because the other sizes were too big. I haven't bought this size shirt since I was a young teenager. The clothing industry seems to be flattering our egos by adjusting the "sizes" so that we think we are trimmer and thinner than we actually are.

In fact, I have seen news stories of clothing stores putting mirrors in their dressing rooms that make you look thinner. Maybe I need to trade in my mirror for one of those! But wait! The British study showed that I don't need such a mirror. I already *think* that I am thinner.

The "body acceptance movement" was blamed for the results of the study.

Size matters

A few years ago, I visited a traveling exhibition that passed through town that showcased actual human bodies that had been preserved through a process called plastination. These bodies were dissected to display various bodily systems and organs. I remember leaving the exhibition feeling a deep reverence for the complexity of the human body. I was also shocked at how small the internal organs of the body actually are. Many of them can be held in the palm of your hand, yet each provides an incredibly important function in the body. Your kidneys, for example, are only about the size of your fist, but they have about one million nephrons in them that filter out liquids and toxic wastes, cleaning your blood up to 300 times a day.

When I saw how small these organs, blood vessels, and nerves were, I realized how easy it would be to overwhelm and damage them by eating platefuls of "Frankenfoods" (fast foods, junk foods, and processed foods) that are digested into substances that effectively choke them instead of energize them, starve them instead of feed them, impair them instead of enable them, and damage them instead of protect them. These tiny organs hardly stand a chance against a body owner who eats massive amounts of junk food day-in-and-day-out, thereby depriving them of the micronutrients (the antioxidants and phytonutrients) they so desperately need and subjecting them instead to micronutrient-deficient foods with harmful ingredients. In fact, it is amazing that our organs can hang in there for as long as they do against such nutritional abuse.

Perhaps we visualize our organs as larger than life, like superheroes who can overcome any odds and push through any opposition to save our skins with their special powers. Maybe if we held these organs in the palm of our hand, saw them struggling to perform their functions within our body, or saw them in an exhibition like the one I attended, we would treat them with greater respect and admiration and eat things that nourish them and do them no harm. For example, if we could see up-close just how small the insides of our arteries are, we might be less inclined to load up our plates with hefty portions of meat, dairy products, and eggs that are full of cholesterol and highly saturated fat that stiffen our arteries, build up plaque, and lead to strokes, dementia, and heart attacks.

So, give the organs of your body a break. Treat them with the respect they deserve. Just say "no" to Frankenfoods and "yes" to whole, plant-based foods.

Eat more, weigh less

Nutritional scientists created the term "energy density" as a measure of calories to weight of various foods. In general, plant-based foods are *low* in energy density, which is a good thing for avoiding unwanted weight gain. Indeed, some studies have shown that those who eat a diet of low energy density foods actually lose weight while eating more and having the same satisfaction from eating. How can that be?

For one thing, plant foods are packed with fiber, which fills up your stomach sooner and helps you feel full faster. Plant foods are also loaded with phytonutrients and other micronutrients that deeply nourish your cells and quench "toxic" hunger (to use Dr. Joel Fuhrman's term), which drives further eating. Finally, because plant foods are full of water and fiber, they are bulky. They take significantly more time to eat, giving you more "chewing time" and culinary satisfaction.

To learn more about this topic, watch Dr. Michael Greger's short video, "Eating More to Weigh Less," on his website at nutritionfacts.org that explains how you can eat more, weigh less, and have better health while doing so.

What you should feed your gut flora

According to Dr. Michael Greger, you have trillions of microorganisms living inside you. Most of them reside in your gut and are sometimes referred to as your *gut flora*. Your gut flora, sometimes called the "forgotten organ," are important to your immune system, digestion, the creation of certain vitamins, and the suppression of potential pathogens, among other things.

Your gut flora come in two varieties: good and bad. When you eat, you are not just feeding your body. You are feeding the one to two pounds of gut flora that live inside your body. Animal foods—including animal fat, cholesterol, and animal protein—establish and feed the bad gut bacteria, while plant-based foods, which are full of fiber, pre-biotics, and other important components, feed and establish the good gut bacteria. When the bad microorganisms flourish, they release carcinogens, produce toxins, and cause digestive problems and infections. They are associated with an increased risk of colon cancer, our second leading cause of cancer death (see

Dr. Michael Greger's videos entitled, "What's Your Gut Microbiome Enterotype" and "Microbiome: The Inside Story," on nutritionfacts.org).

If you eat meat, for example, you are summoning the bad bacteria in your gut that eats meat. That bad bacteria turns that meat into a molecule called TMA (trimethylamine). Your liver then converts TMA into TMA oxide (TMAO). That is a dangerous molecule that drives cholesterol into the artery walls and, according to Rip Esselstyn, is a stronger predictor of heart disease than high blood pressure, smoking, or even *cholesterol* (See Rip Esselstyn's book, *My Beef with Meat*).

What is good nutrition?

Our culture has trained us to think of nutrition as a matter of focusing on a certain set of *macronutrients* in our diet: protein, carbohydrates, fats, minerals, and vitamins. The processed food industry has capitalized on this by telling us over the years that we need more protein, less fat, less gluten, fewer carbs, more vitamins, more calcium (milk), or more fish oil supplements—initiating huge marketing campaigns that often last for years until the current trend waxes old and a new campaign is launched.

What scientists are finding out today is that this approach to nutrition is flawed. Foods in their natural state are not just a collection of a few isolated macronutrients. Nature has packaged them with hundreds of *micronutrients*, such as antioxidants, soluble and insoluble fiber, and phytochemicals or phytonutrients—many of which have not yet even been identified. These micronutrients nourish our cells, affect how our food is absorbed and digested, neutralize free radicals (harmful molecules that are by-products of metabolism), and help fight cancer and disease. They work in synergy—the effect of the entire collection of micronutrients is greater than the sum of the individual components. When natural foods are refined, processed, and stripped of all but a few macronutrients, these other beneficial micronutrients are lost.

The body is much more complex than any of us realize. Its nutritional requirements are complex. We need to think of good nutrition as eating a *variety* of whole, plant-based foods so that we get all of the micronutrients that humans need. Good nutrition is not just "getting enough protein every day" (as marketers have led us to believe) but eating a variety of whole foods *and* the avoidance of processed foods, fast foods, junk foods, and other unhealthy foods, such as of meat, dairy, and eggs (more to be said about these later).

So, contrary to the marketing messages, good nutrition is *not* made up of a small handful of isolated macronutrients that we are told we must juggle in certain proportions for optimal health. That has been the message the processed food industry has pushed for years. It simply is *not* true.

WEEK 7

"Don't let those junk food desires be victorious!"

What does "zero sugar" really mean?

On my way back from a recent hike in the mountains, I pulled up behind a bus at a stop light that had a large advertisement painted on the back that touted a major soda maker's new soda that included the words "zero sugar" in the name of the product. People might think, "Oh, how great! Now it has no sugar, and too much sugar is bad!" But don't be tricked. As far as I could tell from checking out the ingredients listing on its website, it appears that they just changed the name of the product and perhaps tweaked their formula so they could label it differently. The new version still lists aspartame as one of the ingredients. So instead of using the word "diet" in their product name, they now use the words "zero sugar."

This is one of marketers' oldest tricks—pasting a new name or label over the old and keeping the product the same or modifying it only slightly. The assumption is that people can now feel good again about drinking or eating their product because of its new name. I noticed that another major soda maker did the same thing with their diet soda. Marketers get paid a lot of money to come up with these schemes to circumvent people's negative perceptions in a changing cultural environment.

I also heard on the national news recently a news report that drinking diet sodas makes you hungrier and influences you to eat more and put on more weight. They said that you are probably better off drinking soda with real sugar in it than soda with artificial sweeteners. Of course, your best bet is to avoid soda altogether and drink the best thirst quencher on the planet—water—but that is not what the marketers want you to do.

Are chips labeled as "veggie chips" really made from veggies?

While watching the morning news on TV while eating breakfast, I heard a story about a food industry show going on in New York City. The reporter proudly talked about some of the latest trends in the food industry for manufacturing "healthier" foods. The two examples given were cauliflower pretzels and cauliflower chips ("cauliflower" is the new "kale," according to the reporter). But wait a minute. Does adding a bit of ground up cauliflower to a pretzel that is heavily salted make it healthy? Or does making a chip from cauliflower flour, frying it in oil, and dousing it with salt mean it is healthy? Of course not.

The food industry is sensing that more and more people are learning about the value of eating fruits and vegetables and therefore want to eat healthier. So they are making slight adjustments to their otherwise unhealthy ingredients, often by adding small or trivial amounts of dried fruits or vegetables and then putting messages on their packaging to make us *feel* like their product is healthy. It's all about the *feeling*, not the *reality*.

If you don't believe me, go down the chip aisle in the grocery store, pick up a bag of chips marketed as "vegetable" chips, and read the ingredients and nutritional labels. The ingredients label on one bag revealed that they appear to be potato chips with a little tomato paste, beetroot powder, and spinach powder mixed in or sprayed on before they were fried in oil. They still have 290 mg of salt per serving and a measly 1 gram of fiber. Almost half of the calories come from fat—60 out of 130!

But the advertising proudly boasts that they are "veggie chips" that were made with "sea salt" and are "100% natural" and have "30% less fat." It's got to be healthy based on those words and catch phrases, right? Before you believe the marketing hype on the front of the package, read the ingredients and the Nutrition Facts label on the back to get the real story.

Who's watching out for the health of our children?

In the documentary *Fed Up*, Katie Couric discusses one of our society's saddest and most disturbing health issues. Our children are becoming increasingly obese at an alarming rate and suffering serious health consequences as a result, such as fatty liver disease, Type 2 diabetes, increased rates of cancer, a build-up of plaque in their arteries as early as age 10, and other related metabolic and non-metabolic health issues. She reports that in 1980, cases of Type 2 diabetes among adolescents was zero. The number in 2010 was 57,638. At the current rate, by 2050, *one in three* Americans will have diabetes.

But the food industry is not all to blame. We ourselves unwittingly get our children hooked on sugar from a very young age by *giving* them junk food such as packaged breakfast cereals, sodas, cookies, cakes, yogurt (which is full of added sugar), ice cream, and candy. And parents and teachers use candy and treats as the "universal" reward.

Sugary treats are not the only thing of concern. We also give our children lots of highly refined carbs in the form of crackers, white bread, white rice, white pasta, chips, and other highly processed foods in boxes and cans. The carbs in these foods might as well be pure sugar because they have been stripped of fiber and other nutrients so that they are quickly broken down into sugar in our children's digestive tracts where they rapidly enter their blood stream and cause a spike in their blood sugar and a corresponding insulin response.

On top of highly sugary foods and highly refined carbs, we give our children processed meat such as bacon, ham, pepperoni, cold cuts, deli slices (luncheon meat), hot dogs, and sausage—all of which the World Health Organization has classified as Group 1 carcinogens—in the same group as cigarettes, plutonium, and asbestos! We feed our children hamburgers and other red meat on a regular basis, which are classified as Group 2 carcinogens. Did you know that one out of every four deaths in the U.S. is due to cancer?

And how have we allowed our public school lunches to be taken over by the corporate fast food giants? According to Couric's documentary, in 2006, 80 percent of all high schools operated on exclusive contracts with soda companies? By 2012, more than *half* of all U.S. school districts served fast food. When I asked my grandkids what they ate for school lunch while they were here, I frequently heard them report that they ate pizza, French fries, hot dogs, hamburgers, chocolate milk, cookies, and soda. This is not the school lunch I grew up on.

Apart from how unhealthy all this "food" is and the toll it takes on the health of our children, there is another concern that is just as alarming. Children consume very little food to begin with. When all they eat is junk, *where are they going to get the nutrition*? Without nutrition—especially micronutrients like fiber, antioxidants, and phytochemicals that are found only in plant food—there is stunted growth, impaired health, and a greatly increased risk of serious disease.

Because children eat so little food, it is even more important for them to eat healthily. Junk food kills children's appetite for anything else, including healthy food. If you don't believe it, let your children eat junk food in-between meals and then see what they are willing to eat at mealtime.

Parents who take the easy road of letting their children eat whatever they want without proper oversight may not see any immediate consequences in the lives of their children, but statistically, serious consequences will follow, often in the prime of their lives when they need their health to raise their own families, earn a living, and enjoy life.

The tragedy is, it is the children who will suffer for the sins of the parents. Children are too young to be responsible for their own health. Parents must take responsibility for the health of their children. They cannot push that responsibility onto society, the food industry, the government, or anyone else. Our future and the future of our children depend on it.

What's a medium French fry worth?

Here's something to consider: One medium French fry from a popular fast food franchise has 340 calories. 43 percent of those calories come from the fat. To burn off that number of calories, you'd have to:

- Do 1 hour and 6 minutes of light to moderate calisthenics,
- Run 37 minutes at 5 mph
- Snow ski for 42 to 60 minutes
- Vigorously swim laps for 30 minutes, or
- Do light-to-moderate weight lifting for 1 hour and 38 minutes.

And that's if you could somehow burn off the fat in the fries before it was stored as fat in your body, where it is *much* more difficult to burn, as we all know. Remember, "the fat you eat is the fat your wear."

Wake up, America

On the national news recently, they reported that there has been a 43 percent increase in the occurrence of liver cancer in the past 16 years. Livers don't just grow on trees. If you get liver cancer or liver disease and need a transplant, it can be very difficult to find a donor, if you even qualify for a transplant, not to mention the cost.

I often wonder how it is that here in America we can continue to hear one report after another about how disease is skyrocketing and our health is plummeting, yet we largely continue to act as if there is nothing we can do about it. According to a March 13, 2018 ABC news report of a Harvard study, the U.S. spends more on health care than other countries, but we don't fare any better—for example, our life expectancy is shorter and obesity is higher.

It is not the amount of money we are spending on health care that is to blame for these trends.

When we hear about non-health-related problems in society, we expect politicians and professionals to investigate to identify the cause of the problem so we can prevent the problem from occurring again. But when it comes to the ever-increasing trends in disease, we have allowed blinders to be put over our eyes. We have been taught that these trends are just due to the aging population, bad luck, pollution, or bad genes, or we close the blinders entirely and go into denial.

Okay, then. Who helped place those blinders over our eyes in the first place? Could it be:

- The industries that benefit from our being sick, such as the medical profession itself, which focuses on treatment, not prevention; drug companies (big pharma), which make billions of dollars off of cancer drugs alone; and the medical device manufacturing industry?
- The industries that sell the products that we eat that, consumed over time, are linked to serious disease, such as the processed food industry and the meat, dairy, and egg industries?
- Politicians who have sold out to the most powerful lobbyists in the country?

These groups do not want the products they sell threatened or their campaign funds threatened, just like the tobacco and cigarette companies didn't want the products they sold threatened.

The question for us is, "How many alarming news reports do we need to hear before we start asking *what* is causing these trends and *what* we can do to prevent disease *before* we get sick?" The companies that stand to benefit financially in maintaining a sick American population are saying, "Show me the proof—you can't be sure what the cause is." That is exactly the playbook that the big tobacco companies used for decades. Create just enough doubt to put up a smokescreen. After thousands of correlational studies linking smoking with cancer, the government finally agreed, but not until after countless people worldwide had already died from using their product and the companies had made billions.

Today, that smokescreen is becoming increasingly thin with the amount of nutrition research that is piling up—research that shows that eating a whole-food, plant-based diet that avoids highly processed foods, junk foods, meat, dairy, and eggs is likely the healthiest diet on the planet.

What can you do about this situation besides voice your concerns to your elected politicians? Vote with your pocketbook. Stop buying junk. Plunging profits have a way of getting large companies and organizations to think about changing direction and open the door for entrepreneurs to step in and fill the gaps.

Diagnosis: "Unknown"

Do you believe that regardless of whatever medical problem you might have, the medical profession has the tools, techniques, knowledge, and expertise to diagnose your problem? Then maybe you had better think again. Even something as simple as determining the cause of recurring headaches can elude even the best medical professionals with their CT and MRI scans, glucose monitoring studies, sleep studies, blood work, environmental investigations, drug interventions, and other tests and procedures.

Do you also believe that your primary care physician will be the one to champion your cause and persist until a diagnosis is found, like Dr. Gregory House in the TV series *House, M.D.*? Sadly, the opposite is often the case. Patients are the ones who typically have to push their physicians to not give up when a problem does not easily fall into a well-known diagnostic category.

After all, patients are just a ten- or fifteen-minute time slot in a single workday of a doctor, which is not much mental analysis time or effort on the part of the physician. Who has not had to insist on more tests, suggest additional possible causes, ask to see other specialists, and perform research on their own? Even with the patient's prodding, doctors might not be successful in finding the cause of the condition or be able to find a successful treatment.

We sometimes criticize others for putting "blind faith" in a person, organization, or cause, but do we have "blind faith" that the medical profession can help us no matter what our medical issue is?

What we need today is not more "blind faith" in the medical profession, but more individual responsibility for eating healthily so we don't have to diagnose problems in the first place. While not every medical problem or issue can be prevented through diet, many can, and the odds for getting others can be greatly reduced (see Dr. Michael Greger's book, *How Not to Die*).

An intervention with zero side effects

A major news magazine article recently reported that three drug companies recalled their medications over concerns they may contain an impurity, NDMA, which is a possible human carcinogen that could lead to cancer. That sounds pretty shocking—a medicine that is supposed to help you might actually lead to a gruesome death? That is, until you watch the evening news and listen to the ads for medications that air during commercial breaks. These ads show pleasant video snippets of people enjoying life's happiest moments while the narrator runs through a litany of possible side effects that often includes things like cancer, heart attack, stroke, and even death. One of the most puzzling to me is "Don't use this product if you are allergic to it." How would I know if I am allergic to it before I take it? Often, the verbal rehearsal of the possible side effects takes longer than the pitch for the drug itself.

So, let's see. I get this one benefit, but in turn, I must risk incurring side effects that are a mile long that may include serious injury to my health and even death. Hmmm. Just the fact that these commercials are frequent and airing during expensive prime time tells me two things:

- The drug companies are making a lot of money from these drugs to afford this kind of advertising, which means the drugs must be pricey for consumers and health insurance companies, and
- Americans must be suffering from the diseases the drugs are targeting in sufficiently high numbers to justify the cost of the ads.

Have you done a mental check recently on how many ads on TV have to do with selling medications, weight loss pills and programs, and cosmetic weight-loss surgery? I cringe every time I hear a warbling testimonial in one of those ads touting "I just didn't think I could get there, and look at me now" from a person who underwent a surgeon's knife in what had to be major surgery for weight loss. The sad thing is, the surgery did not remove the *cause* of the person's weight gain. I wonder what the person looked like a year or two later. Perhaps a better question is, how did we get to the point in society where someone is so desperate to have "an ideal figure" that they are willing to undergo major surgery in a last-ditch effort to do so? We should be emphasizing good health—not an ideal figure—in our society.

I live in a little suburbia south of a major city. During the last couple of years, there has been a massive expansion at our local hospital. Two huge high-rise buildings have gone up in addition to several new wings that take up almost a city block. When I look out from my second-story deck toward the city, the hospital buildings a mile away rival the skyline of the downtown complex two miles away. I told my wife, "They must be expecting a lot of sick people to support the cost of constructing and staffing those massive new hospital towers."

Sadly, the answer to that supposition is "yes." A recent news article reports that the U.S. cannot keep up with the demand for nurses and doctors. More and more people are becoming sick and need services; hence, the building boom in my little town for a massive new medical complex.

Almost a year ago, after being on a healthy plant-based nutritarian diet for over a year, I went in for my annual physical. The results were outstanding on all measures. Not only had I lost 45 pounds, for a male my age, my annual physical looked more like the one I had when I was in my twenties, all while experiencing zero side effects! Now there's an intervention I can live with!

WEEK 8

"Others are taking notice that you take your health seriously."

Fast food marketers strike again

A major fast food franchise recently announced that they are giving away free medium French fries every Friday for the rest of the year 2018 (I presume in the U.S.) to those patrons who downloaded their app and spent at least $1.00. This is a triple play for them: get more people using their app, where they can send marketing messages directly to you, bring more people into their store, and get more people hooked on their junk food.

French fries is one of those fast foods that combines both fat and sugar (the carbs in the white potatoes are quickly broken down in the digestive tract into sugar), which triggers a stronger response in the addictive pleasure centers of the brain than do either fat or sugar alone. After all, when was the last time you ate just one French fry? Or, how many French fries do you really *want* to eat? Suppliers of legal and non-legal addictive drugs and products use this same technique—give away for free just enough of their product to get the person addicted and you have a paying (albeit addicted) customer for life. Nothing assures a constant stream of income like addiction.

I went to see a blockbuster action movie during the summer at a large mega-movie complex on discount movie night. This huge complex had a lobby that seemed bigger than a Las Vegas luxury casino. Most of it was occupied by a half-dozen or more fast food checkout counters. This was no ordinary theater where popcorn, nachos, soda, and candy were all that was offered. This mega-complex offered name-brand pizza, burritos, hot dogs, hamburgers, chicken fingers, wraps, ice cream cones, a huge soda dispensary island, and a wide assortment of other junk food. Large trays were available that made it convenient to carry your junk-food "meal" right into the theater. Many of the people surrounding me in the theater were feasting on the piles of food they had carried in, sending off a mixture of smells that was quite nauseating.

Another fast food restaurant chain that originally specialized in thinly sliced beef and deli sandwiches has since expanded into offering a variety of other meat sandwiches, which collectively they have made their trademark: A deep-voiced narrator ends every commercial loudly with a marketing jingle about having the meats. I ate at their franchise quite often over the years, not knowing how eating meat was potentially affecting my health. Now, I know that processed meats and red meat have been classified by the World Health Organization as Group I and Group II carcinogens, respectively (the worst categories). Today, I believe their slogan has a limited lifespan. When the general public finally starts to understand the health dangers of eating animal products, that slogan will repel people, not attract them. Maybe the franchise's slogan of the future will be, "We have NO meats!"

The price of modern convenience

Today's commercial enterprises provide products and services that make it convenient for us to do just about anything, including satisfying our hunger. Unfortunately, in doing so, they often compromise the nutritional quality of their products and add ingredients that make us want to buy more.

What if the only thing you could buy in grocery stores were healthy foods? What if, additionally, there were no fast food outlets and restaurants to satisfy your hunger? How would your life change? Would you be in a panic about how you were going to feed yourself and your family three or four times a day? Would your ancestors look down and wonder how their posterity is at a loss to fix real food?

Perhaps this imagined scenario is a good test to see how healthy you are eating. For me, my life would be impacted very little—I would continue preparing my food as usual. But for most Americans, there would be real panic—not just with the food preparation—but with getting themselves, their spouses, and their children to eat real food. The transition from manufactured food to real food is challenging for most people. Perhaps some of you would rather starve to death than switch.

Sound too far-fetched? Perhaps, but during World War II, Nazi-occupied countries like Norway limited what the general population had access to, such as meat, dairy, and eggs, so they could supply troops on the front. The general population had to eat basic staples instead of the food products to which they were accustomed. To the surprise of some investigators, later research showed that the health of these populations actually went up during this period of austerity. After the war was over and people had access to animal products again, overall health went back down and disease rates went back up to their pre-war levels where they continued to rise as the populations became even more "modernized." Of course, animal products may not have been the only factor, but researchers highly suspect it.

No doubt about it. Convenience foods are quick and easy. They require little work, and our brains are programmed to take the path of least effort. These foods are so engineered that the pleasure centers of our brains light up brightly when we eat them. But following the path of convenience does not lead to good health. We must ask ourselves, "Have we sold our health to the god of convenience to satisfy our hunger?"

Have it your way

I heard a commercial for an antacid on TV the other day. They showed a man eating pizza and other acid-producing foods and then relieving his heartburn by taking their product. They ended the commercial with the tag line, "Eat your way," implying that you could continue to stuff your face with these "foods" and then just take a pill to avoid the resulting heartburn.

That commercial is not alone. Other marketing slogans emphasize "having it your way." What I want, I get. This is the era of catering to the consumer's every whim, desire, and fancy. If the consumer wants it, someone will offer it. The marketing messages always follow this logic: "You have the desire? Great! We will satisfy it."

But at what cost? These pitches invariably depict, using every means available to television, the immediate gratification you will have by using their product or service; however, they never mention any long-term negative consequences. Rather, the narrator subtly validates and confirms your desire in the introduction and then offers a product or service that will satisfy it, all without questioning the desire in the first place.

However, just because you want something does not mean that what you want is good for you. There are plenty of bad desires out there in life. People commit crimes, become addicts, destroy families, and do many other terrible things because they want the wrong things and then act on those desires.

Perhaps the man feasting on pizza should consider not just the short-term consequences of his actions—the heartburn resulting from his dietary selection—but the long-term consequences, such as the damage to his health from eating cheese, processed meats, and saturated fats, and the damage to his digestive tract.

So, have it your way, but understand that your way may eventually lead to early heart disease, Type 2 diabetes, cancer, stroke, liver disease, kidney disease, and other metabolic and non-metabolic health disorders. It might even lead to an untimely death.

I like having it my way, but my way is to eat nutritious foods that will maximize my chances of leading a long, healthy, and vibrant life. I hope you will too.

Americans now have almost constantly elevated insulin levels

I recently read an article quoting a local university professor of physiology and developmental biology about the foods we eat. One of his insights was that insulin resistance has become the *most common disorder* in the world and that people's diets ensured that they have almost *constantly elevated* insulin levels. When I heard that, it made a lot of sense. The American diet is made up of around 80 percent processed foods (including junk foods). Most processed foods contain highly processed carbs—sugar, white flour, white rice, white bread, white potatoes, and the like. These foods all spike blood sugar levels and force our bodies to release insulin to lower our blood sugar. But the cells that produce and respond to insulin eventually fail from repeated abuse, resulting in type 2 diabetes.

What would a space alien who was sent to earth to observe our dietary habits record on his futuristic electronic device? Kids eating breakfasts consisting of milk (which is high in sugar itself) poured over highly processed sugar-coated cereals. Lunches consisting of white sandwich bread, processed meats, mayonnaise, and cans of flavored pasta or chicken noodle soup. Dinners consisting of pizza, soda, and garlic breadsticks made with white flour. Adults snacking on chips and candy and drinking sports drinks and soda throughout the day. And families devouring evening treats of ice cream, cookies, cakes, and other desserts. All these foods are full of highly processed carbs and animal products which are linked to high blood sugar and ill health. It's no wonder that our modern dietary habits ensure people have almost constantly elevated insulin levels—they are *constantly* eating processed foods, fast foods, and junk foods!

This is *not* what people want to hear—bad news about what they are eating—so the message and the messengers are ignored or ridiculed. But we cannot ignore the consequences. Predictions are that by the year 2050, 1 in 3 Americans will have type 2 diabetes. That's *one third* of all Americans, including many children and teens. I hope one of them is not you, your

spouse, or one of your children. Countless others will be pre-diabetic and suffer from fatty liver disease.

How long can we deny the hard facts and think that we can set aside basic laws of health both individually and as a country without any serious consequences? How much unnecessary suffering, diminished lives, and expense will this and future generations incur? It wasn't until the government started putting warning labels on cigarette packages that people started waking up to the dangers of smoking. We can be smarter than that.

Another example of a marketing slight-of-hand

A local grocery store chain known for selling healthy fruits and vegetables also sells food masquerading as healthy food. I came across this example during my last shopping trip: "sweet potato tortilla chips." The picture on the front showed slices of sweet potatoes morphing into chips, strongly suggesting that the chips were made from *whole, sliced* sweet potatoes. A quick read on the back revealed that this was not the case. The ingredients label showed they were largely made from—not sweet potatoes—but *stone-ground corn*. Sweet potatoes (dried and otherwise) were shown near the bottom of the ingredients list, just ahead of salt. So just enough sweet potato was sprayed on or added into the mix to make the distorted marketing claim that the product title strongly suggested. Cooking oil was the second ingredient, right after the corn.

A review of the Nutrition Facts label on the back revealed that the product had a lot of fat and highly processed carbs and very little fiber or protein. Nevertheless, the marketing hype on the front had all the right messages: "Sweet potato" (a known healthy superfood, in large type), "Non GMO," "Gluten Free," "0 Trans Fat," "No artificial flavors or preservatives." And, it was being sold in a store known for selling healthy food. So, it's got to be healthy, right? Let's throw it in the cart. No, better to pass.

Once again, here is a product that uses all the latest "healthy food" buzz-terms to relabel and slightly tweak an old product (corn chips) to make it sound healthier. Of course, they will argue that a sprinkling or smidgeon of sweet potato flour does indeed make it healthier. Maybe, but not by much.

Always look at the ingredients listing and the Nutrition Facts label on the package to learn the real story.

Losing weight is not the goal

When people decide to improve their health, the first thing they want to do is lose weight. So, they find a popular diet, or they just begin to starve themselves. After dieting for a number of days, weeks, or months, they realize they cannot adhere to the diet any longer because of hunger, feelings of deprivation, or costs. After going off the diet, they then regain the lost weight over the next several months. This yo-yo dieting batters their self-esteem and damages their health (see Dr. Joel Fuhrman's book, *The End of Dieting*).

But health is far more than physical appearance or how much we weigh. Health comes from the inside out as we eat wholesome foods, exercise, manage stress, and get adequate sleep. Our goal should be to achieve *superior health*, not to lose a fixed number of pounds or inches around our waistline.

If your goal is superior health, you will choose foods that promote *health*, not just *pleasure*. If you are overweight, by eating a healthy diet, you will lose weight, but it will occur naturally, without counting calories and without feeling hungry, and the weight you lose will stay off for good. Ideal weight is a side-effect of healthy eating and living, not the underlying cause of good health.

Are fast food coupons really a bargain?

I don't know about you, but every week I get a collection of newspaper-ad inserts in my mailbox which seem to quickly fill up my waste basket. This stack of glossy ads includes many pages of coupons for fast food and other restaurants. Several restaurants have their own full-page or multi-page brochure. Coupons are all over the place. Buy one, get one free. Take a dollar off here, two dollars off there. Buy this and get that for free. It's almost as if they were giving away free junk food.

If you are not particular about the food you put into your body, you might think this is a real bargain. I know. I was one of those people who used to clip and use these coupons regularly to satisfy my hunger.

But are these coupons real bargains? So it seems on face value, but in the long run, I believe we *pay dearly* for them when we consume fast foods on a regular basis, as most Americans do. Ironically, the real financial payoff doesn't go to the fast food restaurants, who may increase business slightly, but to the doctors, hospitals, drug companies, medical device makers, and others who reap a windfall when we don't take care of our health. Poor health brought on by fast foods may not come tomorrow, next week, or even next year. But those who stand to make a profit wait patiently. They know you will come—eventually.

Society pays in other ways when fast foods (including highly processed foods in the grocery store) become our primary source of calories, as is now the case in America. Dr. Joel Fuhrman has written an outstanding book on that very subject (see *Fast Food Genocide: How Processed Food Is Killing Us and What We Can Do About It*).

What I find hopeful, though, is that people seem to be getting more interested in healthy eating, as evidenced by the marketing messages appearing on processed food packages, more frequent news reports on health-related studies, and more books on nutrition and healthy eating that make the New York Times Bestseller List. The truth has a way of eventually coming forward, as long as we live in a free society and there are people who are interested in knowing it.

WEEK 9

"Keep improving your diet. Strive for progress, not perfection!"

The profession unlikely to go the way of the buggy whip maker

I recently saw a documentary in which a British anthropologist held up a couple of human skulls, one with relatively perfect teeth and the other with missing and damaged teeth. He said that before the arrival of refined sugar in the world, the skulls had intact teeth with little tooth decay. After the arrival of refined sugar, the skulls had extensive missing or damaged teeth and teeth with cavities. In fact, scientists who used CAT scans to examine the remains of ancient Romans who were buried in the eruption of Mount Vesuvius in AD 79 discovered that they had perfect teeth, thanks to a healthy low-sugar diet.

As reported by a recent major newspaper, a team of researchers at the University of North Carolina found that 68 percent of processed foods in grocery stores have added sugar. The article lists over 75 words for "sugar" that are used in ingredients listings and about 60 'juice concentrates' that really are full of "sugar." It's no wonder that Americans have no idea that sugar has been added to just about everything that they buy in the grocery store. The article mentioned that high sugar consumption is linked to obesity, type 2 diabetes, and tooth decay.

In 2018, Americans bought 600 million pounds of candy for Halloween. I'm sure this exceeded the amount of candy that is needed to keep every dentist in the U.S. in business for the foreseeable future. Unfortunately, excess sugar has been linked to a number of other, more serious diseases—not just to dental loss and decay.

The eat-all-you-want diet in which people lose weight

In studies done on a healthy eating program called CHIP (Complete Health Improvement Program), volunteers were given knowledge about healthy eating and then told to eat what they wanted—no portion control, calorie restrictions, or other restrictions were imposed. Instead, they watched videos on whole-food, plant-based eating and were given encouragement and social support to eat healthily.

Six weeks later at the end of the study, participants were eating on average 339 less calories a day because they were choosing healthier foods. They also showed improved results on a number of health and mental health measures. A follow-up done 18 months after the start of the study showed that they were still eating 400 less calories a day! That is the power of sound nutritional education.

As Hans Diehl, founder of CHIP, explains it, "We [as a society] are largely at the mercy of powerful and manipulative marketing forces that basically tell us what to...eat....Everywhere we look, we're being seduced to the 'good life' as marketers define it,...[b]ut this so-called 'good life' has produced in this country an avalanche of morbidity and mortality" (as quoted in Dr. Michael Greger's video, "CHIP: The Complete Health Improvement Program," on nutritionfacts.org).

Why taking a vitamin B-12 supplement is critical for those who don't eat animal products

Vitamin B-12 is an essential vitamin. Your body cannot make vitamin B-12, and it is not found in plant foods. Animals can't make it either. Instead, it is made by micro-organisms found in the soil, which the animals eat when they ingest their food. So if you don't eat animal products, such as meat, you must get it from vitamin supplements or from B-12 fortified food products, such as B-12 fortified almond milk or breakfast cereals.

According to the National Institutes of Health, "Vitamin B12 deficiency is characterized by megaloblastic anemia [which produces abnormal and too few red blood cells], fatigue, weakness, constipation, loss of appetite, and weight loss. Neurological changes, such as numbness and tingling in the hands and feet, can also occur. Additional symptoms of vitamin B12 deficiency include difficulty maintaining balance, depression, confusion, dementia, poor memory, and soreness of the mouth or tongue" (see ods.od.nih.gov).

To avoid these health issues, if you:

- Are vegetarian, vegan, or a nutritarian, or
- Do not otherwise eat meat, or
- Do not regularly eat food products which are fortified with vitamin B-12, then you should probably take a vitamin B-12 supplement, after consulting with your health professional.

Many vitamin B-12 supplements are taken sublingually, by letting the tablet slowly dissolve under your tongue. These supplements are inexpensive, costing only a few dollars for a year's supply.

Note that, if you are taking medications, the NIH website further explains that "Vitamin B12 has the potential to interact with certain medications. In addition, several types of medications might adversely affect vitamin B-12 levels. A few examples are provided below [see the article]. Individuals taking these and other medications on a regular basis should discuss their vitamin B12 status with their healthcare providers."

You can be easily tested for vitamin B-12 as part of the blood lab work that is performed at your annual physical to be sure you are not deficient in this vitamin. When I was tested after a year of eating no meat and taking a regular vitamin B-12 supplement, my vitamin B-12 level was well within the normal range.

Is sweet potato the latest fad in crackers and chips?

Having written previously about sweet potato *chips*, I recently came across sweet potato *crackers* at the store. After this caught my eye, I naturally had to look on the back of the box to analyze the ingredients listing and Nutrition Facts. Once again, the main ingredient was not sweet potatoes, but "organic stone ground yellow corn." These are *corn* crackers more than they are *sweet potato* crackers. At least the next ingredient was sweet potato, just ahead of vegetable oil. The rest of the ingredients were promising though (except the salt): organic flax seeds, organic black sesame seeds, organic chia seeds, sea salt, water, and trace of lime.

After looking over the ingredients, it was time to look at the Nutrition Facts label. Almost half of the calories come from fat (43 percent) which itself makes this an unhealthy snack in my eyes. These crackers are mostly fat-laden corn meal, with some sweet potato mixed in! Sodium (salt) was only 50mg, which is not bad for a cracker or chip. However, there was very little fiber at 2 grams. At least they were low in sugar at 2 grams (apparently, they contain no added sugar, which is good). So all in all, if you don't mind eating mainly fat-laden corn meal, you are good to go. It does have a little sweet potato and healthy seeds mixed in, which is better than many crackers. But for me, I don't want to eat any processed food, especially one that is 43 percent fat calories. Remember, "the fat you eat is the fat your wear."

Again, the front of the box had all the right marketing messages to get you to buy it—"USDA organic," "Organic sweet potato [in huge letters]," "Gluten free," "Flaxseed, sesame, and chia," and "Non-GMO project verified." Sounds like it passed a lot of careful scrutiny by the government and other standards-setting organizations, right? Always read the ingredients listing and Nutrition Facts table on the package. Don't be misled by the marketing hype on the front.

Developing a deeper appreciation for natural, whole foods

When I was in college, I went to hear a Vietnam War veteran give a lecture who had been imprisoned for seven years in a Hanoi prison camp. I read the book he wrote about his experience and really wanted to hear what he had to say in person. Aside from the many tortures and atrocities he endured, I remember clearly a statement he made in his presentation. He said he never wanted to go hungry again. After his release and return to the U.S., he stockpiled enough food storage at his home (including whole grains) to feed himself and his family for several years, should there ever be a shortage of food.

I have found that there are two groups of people who truly appreciate food: those who don't have enough to eat, and those who raise the food we eat. The former group appreciates food because they have too little of it. If you want to better understand how they feel, try fasting for 24 hours, if you are medically able. The second group appreciates food because they know firsthand just how difficult it is to grow.

My dad grew up on a farm and arose very early in the morning for a long, hard day of manual labor. After he left home, got married, and graduated from college, he had seven children over the next several years, of which I was the youngest. As a young child, I remember watching my dad tend to a large orchard and garden of his own to help feed his family, in addition to working a full time job as a chemist and building a house for his family. Although I took part in the planting, weeding, and watering of the garden and the irrigation of the orchard, I was too young to know how much expertise was required to get a plentiful harvest. After I married and finished college, I moved away from my home state for the next 30 years, and, unfortunately, my dad passed away soon after I moved back.

Since then, I have tried growing a much smaller garden of my own. I wish my dad were still around to pass on his comprehensive farmer's knowledge on how to grow food. Pests and diseases attacked my plants. Birds flew down and pecked my berries and clipped young tender starts. Some plants didn't produce. Late frosts and the heat of summer took their toll. My irrigation system broke. The blackberry bushes shot out huge new branches high in the air for several feet in every direction, shading out the adjoining strawberry plants and crowding my aisle ways. The neighbor's trees by my back fence grew taller, shading out more of my garden. Weeds grew, plants needed organic fertilizer, and the soil needed regular replenishing with organic compost. During the harvest, fruit and produce had to be tediously hand-picked every few days and then washed, prepared, refrigerated, frozen, or given away. And finally, after the season was over, vines had to be pruned and dead plants pulled up, removed, and taken away. Sound fun or easy?

Notwithstanding all this, every time I pluck a blackberry, strawberry, or tomato off a vine, I feel a deep sense of wonder and gratitude for this delicious, edible fruit and marvel how this gift suddenly appeared on an otherwise plain vine or branch. What a miracle it all is.

Seeing where real food comes from, knowing firsthand how hard it is to grow, and understanding how precious it is helps me want to eat it as nature intended—in its original state—not in a highly processed, stripped-of-nutrients-and-fiber form that stores on grocery store shelves for weeks or months at a time and that doesn't resemble its original form.

Why you should eat breakfast at home

According to a leading consumer magazine, Americans eat roughly one-third of their breakfasts at fast-food and coffee chains. The article reported which menu breakfast items were "more healthy" than others (in my mind, junk is still junk, even if it is slightly less junky), but what grabbed my attention the most was their list of "Breakfast Bombs: These May Blow Your Nutrition Budget in One Sitting."

At the top of their list was one of my old-time favorites (before I knew better): A major fast food restaurant's big breakfast with hotcakes, which weighed in at 1,350 calories, a whopping 65 grams of fat, and 2,100 grams of sodium! A major bakery chain's spinach and artichoke soufflé (sounds healthy, doesn't it?) came in at 33 grams of fat (19 saturated) and 890 grams of sodium. And finally, a major smoothie franchise's large banana berry classic smoothie registered an amazing 106 grams of natural and added sugars.

With those nutritional facts, isn't it time you set your alarm clock 15 minutes earlier and made a truly healthy breakfast at home?

Is your body slated for "planned obsolescence"?

When I built my house, I tried to choose high-quality, durable materials that would last over a lifetime and provide good, reliable service. I hate products that stop working shortly after I purchase them, that don't perform to expectations, or that don't perform as advertised.

As defined by Wikipedia, "Planned obsolescence is a policy of producing consumer goods that rapidly become obsolete and so require replacing, achieved by frequent changes in design, termination of the supply of spare parts, and the use of non-durable materials." For example, according to an article I recently read in a leading consumer magazine, dishwashers are only made to last about ten years. And old-fashioned incandescent light bulbs were designed to last only a fixed number of hours of illumination, even though they could have easily made them last much longer.

Manufacturers have a lot to gain by building "planned obsolescence" into their products. Consumers have to buy their products again much sooner than they would have otherwise, lifting more money out of their pockets and into the pockets of the manufacturers.

Are we building "planned obsolescence" into our bodies when we eat an unhealthy diet? Absolutely. Research shows that the standard American diet (SAD) leads to the standard American way to an early death (SAWED).

If you don't want your body to be slated for "planned obsolescence," then start eating healthier today!

WEEK 10

"I like the way you are treating your body!"

Why you want the last years of your life to be some of your healthiest

When do you think it is too young for a person to die from a heart attack, cancer, stroke, or other disease? In their 40s, 50s, 60s, 70s, or 80s? When you hear, for example, of someone dying from a heart attack in their 60s, do you think, "That's sad, but not surprising, given that they were 65 years old—they lived a full life"?

As a society, do we expect that death and disease starts in our 50s or 60s and gets worse with each subsequent decade? Do we subscribe to what the British writer Anthony Powell quipped when he said, "Getting old is like being increasingly punished for a crime you didn't commit"? When we are young, do we look at "old age" and equate it with crippling diseases, bent-over postures, shuffling feet, and impaired health?

To bring it a little closer to home, when you reach "old age" (however you defined it when you were, say, in your twenties), do you think you will be ready to resign yourself to a life of chronic pain, doctor visits, healthcare bills, and loss of freedom due to ill health?

As one who, in some people's eyes, has already reached the onset of "old age" (I do qualify for "senior" pricing at many places), I can tell you that when that time comes, you will not want to resign yourself to years or decades of declining health, painful disabilities, and severe physical limitations.

Think about it. When you reach "old age":

- You might find yourself in a situation where your kids are finally out of the house and independent.
- You might be retired or near retirement and thus have more time to pursue goals and activities you previously only dreamed about.
- You might be a grandfather or grandmother and love interacting with your grandchildren, finding joy in being part of their lives.
- You might want to be around to see your grandchildren graduate from school, marry, and have families of their own.
- You might be wiser now than ever before, having wrestled with the challenges of life for many decades.
- You might know firsthand the consequences, good or bad, that follow the choices that you and others have made.
- Your maturity and character might be the best it has ever been.

- Your insight into what builds and strengthens society and humanity might be richer.

So why would you want *this* time in your life—your crowning years—to be crippled by unnecessary bad health or even cut short by a premature death?

Of course, we all age physically as we grow older, which imposes limitations, pain, and ultimately disease and death. But what we are talking about here is *unnecessary*, *avoidable*, or *premature* suffering and disease. Not all suffering and disease in old age is preventable. Some is simply due to the aging process. But certainly some exists which can be avoided or delayed for a number of years, according to nutritional research.

"Old age" may seem like a long way off, but your time will come. Why not make it some of your best years by consistently eating healthily while you are young so you can enjoy maximum health during your senior years, as well as enjoy better health during your younger years? As Kim Williams, former President of the American College of Cardiology, said, when asked why he follows a plant-based diet, "I don't mind dying, I just don't want it to be my fault."

Is your goal to feed your family or nourish your family?

As I walked by the food counter on my way out of a wholesale club the other day, I reviewed the large food-court picture menu high up above the service counter. Pizza, hot dogs, ice cream, soda, and other unhealthy items dominated the scene. The popularity of these items was apparent—a large crowd of people were eating these foods at nearby tables. The low prices, the giant portion sizes, and the convenience seemed to be a main attraction.

Although people on the go are often caught unprepared to feed their families while they are away, I saw some individuals carrying supersized steaming pizza boxes out the door. It made me wonder. Is our goal simply to *fill up* the stomachs of our family as quickly, easily, and as cheaply as possible, or is our goal to *nourish* the bodies of our family with healthy foods and invest in their long-term physical health?

Are we seduced by the inexpensive prices, the convenience, and the speed at which we can buy fast foods and other junk foods to satisfy the hunger pains of our loved ones? Should price, convenience, and speed be the criteria for how we choose to feed our families?

To promote good health, we should consciously evaluate *what* we are feeding our families at every meal. Our goal ought to be to *nourish* our families, not just *feed* them. While it may take more planning, time, and inconvenience to feed them healthy food, think of it as an investment in your most prized possession. After all, parents make huge investments in their children's college education and in their personal development through music lessons, dance lessons, sporting team participation, and other activities. Why would they not invest in their children's health?

We live in a unique time—a time when it is possible to fill our family's stomachs with junk and to do so cheaply. Or, we can fill their stomachs with nutrient-dense, natural foods that will deeply nourish their bodies. The choice is yours.

Don't be afraid to learn about healthy eating

Do you avoid thinking about the topic of healthy eating because you could never see yourself as a full-blown vegetarian or vegan?

The terms "vegetarian" and "vegan" are emotionally charged words. If someone had told me that I would be eating a nutritarian diet (a whole-foods, plant-based diet that also avoids highly processed foods, junk foods, processed oils, and foods with added sugar) in just a few short years, I would have laughed and said that it was impossible. Like most Americans, I thought that vegetarians and vegans were a little strange. I was fully convinced along with other Americans that the standard American diet (SAD) was perfectly healthy. It was only after I was diagnosed with two different deadly cancers within two weeks of each other that I began to reconsider that my paradigm might be out of sync with reality. After that diagnosis, my assessment of my diet was not just an intellectual muse—it was a matter of life and death.

In cognitive terms, labels simplify our lives. They are ways for our minds to judge something and ultimately dismiss the need for more intellectual or unbiased investigation just based on the label alone, thus saving mental energy. If we label something as "tastes poorly," (think "broccoli" or "peas" for many people) then we can dismiss eating it because we have labeled it and can act just based on the label alone.

But what if our labels are incorrect or imperfect? If so, we have misjudged or dismissed something out-of-hand that might in fact help us.

Even if you could never see yourself becoming a full-blown "vegan," "vegetarian," or "nutritarian," do not dismiss your need to learn more about healthy eating or dismiss any consideration about what you can do to eat healthier based on emotionally charged labels. You may never become a vegetarian or vegan. But there is still much you can do to improve your health, even without doing so. The more healthy foods that you eat, the better!

So, add some additional fruits, vegetables, whole grains, beans, or raw nuts to your diet, and avoid going out for fast food just one less time a week. *Everything* you do to eat healthier will have benefit. It is *not* an all-of-none proposition.

Firefighter satisfaction survey

Would you be satisfied if you had a fire in your home and the firefighters simply came in and, *instead* of putting out the fire, replaced the batteries in your smoke detectors so the noise wouldn't keep you awake? Is that what we do when we go to the doctor and get medicine to make the *symptoms* of our health problems go away instead of addressing the causes that set our nutritional house ablaze in the first place?

Do you believe that many of our major health issues could be prevented, reduced, or greatly delayed if only we ate a healthy diet? If not, then it is easy to avoid taking responsibility for your health by chalking up any health problems to bad genes, stress, the environment, bad luck, or simply old age. Certainly those things can contribute to disease, but as Dr. Joel Fuhrman, Dr. Michael Greger, and other nutrition advocates like to say, "You can reshuffle the genetic deck you have been dealt through diet."

By far and away, the greatest influence on most of the major diseases that Americans suffer today is diet. According to some leading cardiologists, for example, heart disease is almost totally *preventable* if only we ate a whole-foods, plant-based diet and got adequate exercise and rest. And, as reported in the massive Global Burden of Disease Study, funded by the Bill and Linda Gates Foundation, the number one dietary risk factor for death and disease worldwide is not eating enough fruit and vegetables.

Perhaps, then, it is time to start taking responsibility for our health by reading Dr. Michael Greger's book, *How Not to Die*, or by listening to his video of the same title on his website, nutritionfacts.org, that explains how diet can help prevent the top 15 causes of death in America.

Plant-based foods power arduous summer hike

Earlier this summer, I climbed a local mountain that rises to 11,101 feet in elevation. I climbed 4,812 vertical feet and about 10 miles in distance. It is listed as a hard hike, and indeed it was.

For food, I took 2 oranges, 2 apples, 3 slices of home-made 100 percent whole wheat bread, a few grapes and blueberries, and a couple of nut bars. I had plenty of energy for the climb just eating fruit, nuts, and whole-wheat bread.

At my age, these hikes are getting a little more challenging, but so far so good. I recover so much faster eating a plant-based diet as well. And I felt better than I expected to feel the next day.

The importance of eating dark, leafy greens every day

A leading consumer magazine apparently joined the "eat yourself healthy" movement in a recent issue's cover story. This issue had ten pages of articles on various topics, including one on fruit and veggie superpowers describing the benefits of eating blueberries, cherries, raspberries, peaches, watermelon, bell peppers, corn, eggplant, tomatoes, and zucchini.

Another article discussed the importance of eating dark, leafy greens, and listed many benefits to eating them, such as slowing cognitive decline, lowering your risk of death from heart disease, and lowering your risk of breast, colon, and pancreatic cancers.

Dr. Michael Greger and Dr. Joel Fuhrman both strongly recommend eating a large salad every day made up of dark, leafy greens (be sure to use an oil-free, homemade salad dressing though, as processed oils are very high in calories per gram, are pure fat, and offer little nutritional value). Although eating a big salad like this every day may sound challenging, you can choose recipes that use leafy greens or just throw a couple of handfuls of greens into your fruit smoothie. You can maximize the absorption of the vitamins and nutrients in your greens by eating a little healthy fat along with them by consuming some nuts, ground up seeds, or some avocado (or guacamole) in the same meal.

Most stores sell pre-washed greens either in a mix or by themselves in bags that make it very convenient to get your daily quota. I buy mine in "bulk" size packages from big box stores. However you eat them, make it a habit to do so daily. Greens are the means to achieving better health!

When the scientific universe collides with popular culture

How do we react when research findings in nutrition go contrary to what is accepted, popular, or even ingrained into our culture? Is our knee-jerk reaction to dismiss the study as flawed, to say it is only an isolated study, or to laugh it off with a joke? This may be a possibility, but what if the findings are replicated across many different studies, researchers, and organizations, especially those who don't have a vested interest in the outcome?

Do you think you could be open-minded and consider changing your lifestyle based on the reported findings? Try this on for size. As reported recently by the news, according to a massive new study of alcohol consumption, no level of drinking alcohol is healthy, and the healthiest thing you can do is to abstain entirely.

The study determined that one third of the population in the world drink alcohol, which led to 2.8 million premature deaths in 2016 and accounted for about 27 percent of cancer deaths in women and 19 percent of cancer deaths in men over age 50. That's between one fourth and one fifth of all cancer deaths in people over the age of 50! That's death at about the same rate (1 in 5) in people who have cancer as people who die from smoking every year today (1 in 5), and smoking has declined from 45 percent of the population in 1954 to about 16 percent in 2014.

We all know that smoking causes cancer. The anti-smoking campaign has been hugely successful. But how many of us know that *alcohol causes cancer*? I cannot even comprehend a number as large as 2.8 million premature deaths.

But doesn't moderate drinking have benefits for your health? Not according to this large meta-analysis.

Was this a single study? Not even close. Researchers looked at 592 studies in 195 countries to produce these findings! This meta-analysis consolidated the findings from almost 600 other studies!

So, are you ready to go stone-cold sober? Do you believe that drinking alcohol causes cancer? If not, what will it take to convince you? 1,000 studies? 10,000 studies?

It took over 7,000 studies to convince the Surgeon General of the United States that smoking caused cancer before he took appropriate action. Unfortunately, countless millions of people had already died or contracted cancer by then, while the tobacco industry grew wealthy.

WEEK 11

"You're definitely not one to go along with the crowd when it comes to taking care of your health!"

Who is cherry picking now?

I have talked to individuals who dismiss the need to eat a whole-food, plant-based diet because they assert that Dr. Joel Fuhrman and Dr. Michael Greger are cherry picking the scientific research and only reporting findings that agree with their dietary philosophy, or they are reporting studies that don't meet the strictest of scientific standards (randomized, double-blind, placebo-controlled studies where one randomly assigned group is forced to eat a certain way and another is left alone and used as a control group).

Aside from the unethical idea of forcing people to eat unhealthily so you can measure the effects of an unhealthy diet, proponents of the cherry picking accusation may have been able to raise some doubts in the past when there were just a few scientific findings with conflicting results. However, today, the accusers are starting to thin out. The numbers of studies showing that a whole-food, plant-based diet is one of the healthiest on the planet has soared. The health benefits of eating more plants, such as fruits, dark-leafy greens, and a variety of other vegetables, is being recognized and reported more frequently by the press, by fitness magazines, and by leading consumer magazines. Both Dr. Greger and Dr. Fuhrman cite numerous peer-reviewed, scientific journal articles in their writings and online postings to substantiate their recommendations.

Who is willing to argue these days that eating more fruits and vegetables does *not* lead to better health? Although eating meat, dairy, and eggs is still a controversial topic—largely because it is so ingrained in our culture and because of the influence and control of those who have a vested financial interest in maintaining the status quo—even that frontier will someday be "discovered" by the general population as well.

With all the evidence available today, I believe it is cherry picking to *disregard* the mainstream body of research and claim that eating the standard American diet is a healthy way of eating.

What neglecting your health can potentially cost you

A news story recently aired about a school teacher in Austin, Texas who had a heart attack and was taken to a hospital where they operated on him and put in several stints. Even though he had health insurance through his teaching job, the hospital was out-of-network, so different limits applied. The insurance only paid $55,000 and the teacher was stuck with paying the remaining $109,000 out of his own pocket. It was only through the unwanted attention and scrutiny of the news story that the hospital felt pressured and finally reduced his bill.

The reporter said that when you go to the hospital, you are at their mercy as far as how much they charge you. All kinds of things are marked up to astronomically high prices. Although they suggested that you try to negotiate a lower bill, how many of us are really equipped to do this, have the knowledge and experience to contest it, or can even read a hospital bill and understand it?

It is far cheaper to eat healthily in the first place to avoid as many medical expenses as you can. If you think eating fresh fruit is expensive, just remember what one procedure in a hospital might cost you. You will never bemoan the cost of eating healthily again. Eating the right foods is an investment in your health and is far cheaper in the long run. If you don't believe it, just wait and see.

"Your kids will love it!"

The other day, I happened to see two news-show hosts enthusiastically talking about the new smaller-sized, sugar-coated donuts that will be offered by two national fast food chains. With all their bright colors and luscious sugar frosting, they did indeed look enticing. As if to put their final stamp of approval on them, they ended the segment with "Your kids will love it."

Should that be the criteria by which I feed my family—my kids will love it? My grandkids love candy, fast food, junk food, and anything else with fat and sugar in it, but eating those foods doesn't lead to good health. Now, parents stopping for one junk food meal can add more junk food item to their dinner table—sugar-coated donuts.

It appears that fast food restaurants are looking for additional ways to increase their revenue by broadening their offerings to include other forms of fast food. This is taking a bad situation and making it even worse.

Children are too young to choose whether to eat healthy food or junk food. If you put junk food in front of them, they will eat it. It is the parent's responsibility to feed their children healthy food and to teach their children how to take responsibility for their own health as they grow up.

It might be rewarding for parents to hear their kids shout grateful approvals when they are served hamburgers and sugar-coated donuts, but is this responsible action on the part of the parents?

The ten most addictive foods in the world (duh!)

A recent study from the University of Michigan identified what they believe are the ten most addictive foods. These are foods that people found hard to put down. It was no surprise to learn that the most addictive foods had two things in common—a high fat content and a high glycemic load (from sugar and refined carbs).

This is consistent with research that shows that fats plus carbs triggers a greater pleasure response in the brain than the sum of the two do alone.

The ten most addictive foods were, in order of most addictive:

1. Pizza
2. Chocolate
3. Chips
4. Cookies
5. Ice cream
6. French fries
7. Cheeseburger
8. Soda (not diet)
9. Cake
10. Cheese

The foods they found the least addictive were cucumbers, carrots, beans without sauce, apples, plain brown rice, broccoli, bananas, salmon, corn without butter or salt, and strawberries. Funny thing—I love all of these least addictive foods (except the salmon).

Define your diet by what you eat, not by what you can't eat

According to the dictionary, a vegan is "a person who does not eat meat or use animal products." According to this definition, you could be a vegan while living solely off of French fries, potato chips, and soda (perhaps this reminds you of a college roommate).

This example demonstrates that a healthy diet cannot be defined solely by what you *can't* eat. This is why Dr. Joel Fuhrman invented the phrase "nutritarian diet" to describe a way of eating that promotes eating a variety of whole, plant-based, *nutrient-dense* foods—whole grains, fruits, vegetables, legumes (especially beans), nuts, and seeds. Although his diet does require that you avoid unhealthy "foods," it focuses on what you *should* be eating every day, not so much on what you *shouldn't* be eating. And to the point, if you ate everything you should be eating, there simply won't be much room left over for the junk you shouldn't eat anyway.

Aside from how a healthy diet should be defined, there are emotional and psychological reasons to avoid focusing on what you shouldn't eat. When you think about all the "treats" you shouldn't eat, the temptation to eat them increases. You begin to feel deprived all over again and wonder why you are not eating them. After all, it's hard not to feel deprived when almost everyone around you is glutting themselves on pizza, cheeseburgers, French fries, ice cream, cookies, chips, donuts, and other junk food with seemingly no immediate health consequences. They appear to be living the "good life" while you aren't, right?

To avoid feeling deprived, focus your mind on the benefits you get from what you *can* eat, not on what you can't eat. Namely, you should:

- Remember that good health cannot be bought—it must be earned through healthy eating.
- Remember how good you feel when you eat healthily and how lousy you feel when you don't. Most people who tune into their bodies know that "when you eat junk, you feel like junk" at some point afterwards.
- Remember that you can't expect people in white coats to undo with surgery, medications, or a few days in the hospital the damage you do to your body from years of unhealthy eating.

- Remember that when you eat healthily, you enjoy a more vibrant, energetic life now and add "bonus" years to your lifespan.
- Remember that by eating the right foods, you dodge future avoidable healthcare costs (consider the teacher in Austin I wrote about who was billed $109,000 after insurance for his brief hospital stay after a heart attack).
- By eating responsibly, you also avoid the pain, suffering, and loss of freedom that comes from disease and health problems and from passing through "one-way doors."
- Remember how good it feels to be regular in the bathroom from all the fiber you are eating.
- Remember how good it feels to keep your waist line exactly where it is with no further expansion.
- Remember how good it feels to keep your energy more level instead of up and down like a yo-yo.
- Remember how good you feel when you respect your body instead of running it into the ground like something that can be easily discarded and replaced.
- Remember all the delicious, whole foods you have waiting for you at home—that fresh peach, slice of watermelon, or bowl of blueberries; that tasty nutritarian entrée; that side dish of brown rice, corn-on-the-cob, lentils, or quinoa; that dish of steamed mixed vegetables; that handful of raw nuts; and that big, dark-green, leafy salad with avocado dressing.

So, the next time you drive by the ice cream store and your mouth starts to water, before your pull in, kick your brain in the amygdala and mentally review this list.

Although nutritarian recipes may not "blow out" the pleasure centers of your brain like sugar and fat (and cocaine) do, they do offer genuine culinary enjoyment, increased eating times, and long-term satisfaction. To be committed, though, you must firmly believe that the long-term benefits are worth the "sacrifice" of turning a blind eye to artificial food.

You really *can't* have your cake and eat it too, which is what many Americans are trying to do. The laws of nature simply won't allow it. What you eat day-in-and-day-out is what largely determines your health, both today and tomorrow.

Another reason to consider giving up eating meat: Meat may contain banned drugs

A recent cover story of a leading consumer magazine asked the question, "What's really in your meat?" According to their own tests, they detected banned drugs in beef, poultry, pork, and turkey. These drugs had antidepressant, anti-inflammatory, antibiotic, or other characteristics.

Their scientists believe that the cut-off levels for these banned drugs established by our own U.S. Agriculture Department's Food Safety and Inspection Service (FSIS) are too liberal, so they established their own cut-off levels that they believe were safer. All of the different types of meat they tested had *some* samples that were above both cut-off levels. They speculated that these substances might be showing up in our meat supply because of improper use in administering drugs to animals, counterfeit drugs, contaminated feed, and intentional misuse.

Note that this article only focused on four drugs. Other investigators have shown that meat samples are sometimes contaminated with other harmful chemicals and bacteria because of the feed the livestock eat, the hormones they are injected with, and the livestock fecal matter that gets onto or into the meat during processing.

Many people believe they *must* eat meat to get enough protein in their diet or to get "all of the essential amino acids they need (the building blocks of protein)." This has been drilled into our heads for years. But that is a myth. The truth is, you can easily meet all your protein needs and get all of your essential amino acids by following Dr. Joel Fuhrman's plant-based nutritarian diet. As one documentary stated, there has never been a documented case of protein deficiency in those eating a plant-based diet when the individuals were eating sufficient calories to sustain life.

Aside from the harmful drugs, chemicals, and bacteria that meat may contain, eating substantial quantities of animal protein, as most Americans do, is suspected by some healthy eating advocates to be linked to the following additional health risks:

- Increases in your risk of cancer, dementia, type 2 diabetes, and heart disease.
- Increased blood cholesterol levels.

- The creation of certain harmful substances when it is digested (such as TMAO, after it has been processed by your gut and liver).
- The stimulation of the production of certain hormones (such as IGF-1).
- Feeding the growth of the "bad" microflora in your intestines.

Moreover, meat has no fiber, whereas plant-based sources of protein have lots of fiber. Because natural fiber is so important to good health, fiber should probably be listed as an essential "nutrient" in our diet, even though it does not provide any calories, the same as other micronutrients that we need. For example, fiber feeds and promotes the growth of the "good" bacteria in your gut, which has been shown to boost your immune system and provide many other beneficial effects to your health, yet 97 percent of Americans do not meet their minimum daily intake of fiber.

Where the good stuff isn't

A national fast-food chain asserts that their franchise is where you can find "the good stuff." Yes, that may be the place where certain pleasure centers of your brain are set all aglow, but if you define "good stuff" as "stuff that is good (healthy) for you (according to the nutritarian definition of what is healthy)," then I believe that this is not where the good stuff is. For that, you have to look to a much less visited, less publicized, and lonely location—the produce section of your local grocery store. Fruits and vegetables are the healthiest and most nutrient-dense foods on the planet.

Are you eating enough fruits and vegetables? Try listing all of the fruits and vegetables you eat on a regular basis. If your list consists of only six or so items, you are not alone. According to a 2009 report by the CDC, only 14 percent of adult Americans eat at least 2 servings of fruit and at least 3 servings of vegetables daily. Adolescents are even worse—only 9.5 percent consume at least 2 servings of fruit and at least 3 servings of vegetables a day.

The protective powers of eating fruits and vegetables is legendary. They reduce your chances for getting cancer, heart disease, dementia, type 2 diabetes, liver disease, kidney disease, and a variety of other diseases, while strengthening your immune system, helping you control your weight, and increasing your chances for a longer life. And eating many fruits is a real treat—they are sweet and so enjoyable. What's not to like?

You would think that with all these benefits, we would be flocking to the produce section of the grocery store in great numbers and that fruits and vegetables would be sold out in no time. If there were a pill you could take that would give you all these benefits with virtually no side effects, how popular do you think it would be? How much would you be willing to pay for it? But we don't need a pill. We just need to eat more fruits and vegetables.

WEEK 12

"Aren't the benefits of healthy eating amazing?"

Want to slow down how fast you age?

Cosmetic and skin care manufacturers make billions selling products that make us look younger and healthier than we really are or that hide the first signs of aging. But appearances can be deceiving, and everyone knows there is no Fountain of Youth. Alright, but is there a way to slow down the aging process, not just cover it up with expensive makeovers?

Apparently, we can—by protecting our telomeres and by hampering the activity of the enzyme TOR in our bodies.

Telomeres protect the end of each strand of DNA that protects our chromosomes, like the plastic coating on the ends of shoelaces. Without them, the DNA strand can become damaged with resulting consequences to cell performance.

We inherit our telomeres from our parents, but regardless of how long they are, they get shorter as we age. In fact, every time our cells divide, they get shorter. The average cell divides 50 to 70 times before it expires.

Research suggests that those with longer telomeres live longer. Eating a plant-based diet has been shown to boost telomerase activity and may even increase the length of telomeres.

It also appears that another enzyme, TOR (target of rapamycin), also contributes to the aging process. Eating more plant-based foods and less animal products has been shown to hamper TOR activity.

Although these are not the only factors that contribute to aging, they appear to play a definite role. Eating a healthy diet has been shown to influence these factors and slow down aging. Here's to staying young!

Why don't people act when they know an impending disaster is coming their way?

At the time of this writing, Hurricane Florence, a major Category 4 hurricane, is approaching the eastern seaboard of the U.S. The authorities ordered a mandatory evacuation of everyone in the affected coastal areas. However, one law enforcement leader stated that 50 percent of the people don't heed the evacuation order and stay put anyway.

I was stunned. I always thought that everyone left except for a few really stubborn souls. A Category 4 hurricane can have winds from 130 to 156 mph. The National Hurricane Center website declares that "Catastrophic damage will occur" for a hurricane of this magnitude. In addition to winds that are as strong as an F2 tornado, storm surges several feet high can sweep in and destroy everything in their path. How can people think that they can hunker down inside a typical American stick-built house and pretend that they will be safe or that all will be well?

Apparently, half of the people do.

If even the immediate threat to their physical safety and a threat to their very lives cannot motivate people to act, then how can we ever hope to motivate others to change the way they eat to avert the personal, social, and national health disasters that await us if we continue to eat the standard American diet?

Many public health officials have warned us, for example, of the impending "tsunami of national debt" our country will face if we do not turn around current disease trends. For example, right now, some researchers estimate that two out of every three Americans are overweight or obese. At the current rate, 95 percent of all Americans will be overweight or obese in two decades. By 2050, 1 in every 3 Americans will have diabetes. This is in addition to the rising rates of heart disease, stroke, cancer, liver disease, kidney disease, Alzheimer's, dementia, and many other diseases and health issues.

Hopefully, you will not ignore real threats that may soon be knocking at your door. Instead, I hope you will voluntarily choose to "evacuate" from any unhealthy ways of eating in your life and ward off avoidable future health disasters by making the change to a whole-food, plant-based diet.

Post note: We all take risks in life, and everyone has their own situation and reasons for doing so. It is sad that sometimes those who would like to leave the target zone of an approaching hurricane feel that they can't because of a fear of the unknown, financial resources, disabilities, lack of transportation, or some other reason. While it is understandable, the threat remains and does not discriminate—sometimes things play out alright and sometimes they don't. I hope that the people in these situations have caring neighbors or family members who are willing to help look after the welfare of their fellow human beings. The rest of us too can support those relief organizations, such as the American Red Cross, that help people in these situations, or we can volunteer our own services if we are able. Since I wrote this article, the hurricane made landfall as a Category 2 hurricane, but because of its size and slow movement, it caused extensive flooding up to a couple of hundred miles inland. Some people died and many more had to be rescued who did not evacuate.

When is a good time to have a heart attack?

On the news recently, they showed a convenience-store surveillance video in which a clerk fell unconscious to the floor from a heart attack after which two young men who had witnessed the collapse then proceeded to rob the cash register and loot the store.

This made me think, is there a good time to have a heart attack? I certainly wouldn't want to have a heart attack when I was driving my family down the freeway at 75 miles per hour, when I was carrying my newborn grandson on my shoulder across our hard tile floors, when I was operating my chainsaw, or when I was walking my two-year-old granddaughter down the sidewalk next to a busy residential street. In these circumstances, my heart attack might not only take my own life, but the lives of other innocent people—loved ones, co-workers, by-standers, or other drivers and their families.

So, having a heart attack is not just about you. It's also about family members and loved ones who will be traumatized by your collapse and possible death, the people who may be injured or killed when you suddenly black out, the volunteers who go out looking for you when you don't return from the mountains, and the medical and other professionals who come to your aid.

A few years ago, while I was out on my morning walk around the neighborhood, I was approached by a terrified young man whose buddy had suddenly collapsed in the adjoining park. He asked if I had a cellphone to call for help. Unfortunately, I had forgotten to charge my phone the previous night, so I had left it plugged in at home. After telling him to go knock on some nearby houses, I ran home and knocked on the door of a neighbor who was an emergency room doctor.

He rushed over to the collapsed young man in the park behind his house and worked on him for almost an hour, even after the ambulance had arrived, as his condition was too critical for him to be transported to the hospital. Unfortunately, he died on the scene despite anything anyone could do for him. His parents, of course, were heartbroken when they found out. It was later determined that this young man had died from a previously unknown health condition, but his sudden collapse and death left all of us emotionally and physically shaken.

In my judgement, there really is no good time to have a heart attack.

If you agree, then what can you do to make sure that "my heart attack day" is unlikely to ever come? Easy—eat a whole-food, plant-based diet and avoid fast food, junk food, processed foods, and animal products. Leading cardiologists have stated that heart disease is a *totally preventable* disease for most Americans. All we have to do is to change what we eat, exercise regularly, and manage stress. Unfortunately, that may be asking too much for some people. They would rather suffer a heart attack or death than change what they eat.

The question we all should ask ourselves every day is this: Is what I am eating *feeding* a future heart attack or *preventing* one?

Why you may want to close your kitchen early every day

Before I became a nutritarian, I looked forward to plunking myself down on the couch every night after playing with my kids to read a book or watch a TV program while I enjoyed one or more treats—chocolate chip cookies, ice cream, chips, cake, buttered popcorn, and the like. It was almost as if I couldn't watch TV or even sit on the couch unless I was eating. This was my reward for the day—an intense period of eating one highly pleasurable food after another. It was a period of self-soothing, or should I say, self-medicating (not too strong of a statement, now that I know how junk food affects the brain).

The only problem was, over time, my waistline expanded, my weight shot up, my cholesterol and blood pressure both went through the roof (requiring medication), I was forced to buy a new wardrobe, and I set myself up for a future health catastrophe, which finally knocked on my door as two kinds of deadly cancer.

Although I stopped eating sugar and junk food for a few years after I was diagnosed with cancer, I gradually slipped back into my old ways. It wasn't until I learned about the benefits of a whole-food, plant-based diet that I fully converted over to healthy eating. But I still loved my evening snacks. I just switched to eating healthy snacks from eating unhealthy ones. At my age, these excess calories made it difficult to keep my weight and waistline exactly where they were.

So, I decided to shut down my kitchen after dinner, which was not a problem because I no longer had small children or teenagers in the house. To help reinforce this nightly closure in my mind, I flossed and brushed my teeth after dinner instead of right before going to bed. This helped me avoid snacking during the rest of the evening, as I really didn't want to go through that ritual again.

Funny, though, I found out that I really can enjoy watching a TV program or reading a book without eating all those treats, and, when the next morning arrives, I am genuinely hungry when I break my fast, or "break-fast."

"Life is too short not to enjoy it."

A chef being interviewed for his new baking show made the statement, "Fun, family, food—life is too short not to enjoy it!" While I agree with his stated intent to enjoy life, I'm not so sure I should be making my "short life" even shorter or sicker by eating unhealthy foods. That phrase seems to be popular among those who want to justify eating or doing anything they want, not just to justify eating an occasional treat.

Some of you might remember a similar philosophy—"You only go around in life once"—that was used in beer commercials for many years to sell beer. Read my prior article, "When the scientific universe collides with popular culture," to know the likely consequences of following that advice.

A careless, irresponsible life is not, in my opinion, a life well lived. I believe that the deeper satisfactions in life come when we improve our character, raise responsible families, serve and build up others, make sustained efforts and sacrifices to achieve worthy goals, and serve God, family, and country. In my mind, a better slogan to follow would be, "Life is too short to throw it away through careless or irresponsible living."

We must remember that what marketers are selling is not the royal road to bliss and "the good life." This was beautifully stated by Hans Diehl, founder of the CHIP program, which I quoted previously but bears repeating here:

"We [as a society] are largely at the mercy of powerful and manipulative marketing forces that basically tell us what to…eat.…Everywhere we look, we're being seduced to the 'good life' as marketers define it,…[b]ut this so-called 'good life' has produced in this country an avalanche of morbidity and mortality."

The problem with diets that have built-in cheat days and cheat foods

The other day, I heard a popular talk show hosted by a well-known TV doctor. He was promoting an almost vegan diet (he does allow some meat) that has a built-in weekly "cheat day" plus two desserts per week and two drinks of alcohol per week. Almost sounds too good to be true—eat what I want one day a week and have desserts and alcohol on two other days (although I personally don't drink alcohol).

To me, this diet really is too good to be true. The doctor promotes this diet as a permanent way of eating 365 days a year for the rest of your life. But is eating unhealthily one day a week and eating a couple of junk foods desserts two other days a week a good compromise? This diet may help some people who are trying to make the transition to a healthy diet, but stopping when you are halfway there and saying that you have "made it" and can now quit is not, in my opinion, a prescription for long-term health.

I guess his reasoning is that an occasional cheat day will not make a huge difference and will help entice and "ease" people over to healthier eating. The problem here is with the definition of "occasional." Occasional is a vague term that can mean anything from every other day to once or twice a year. A whole day of unhealthy eating once a week is not, in my opinion, "occasional." It's like running a marathon and then shooting yourself in the foot. Why would you want to set yourself back one out of every seven days? And who wants to tread water when their goal is to reach the other side?

Now, if later research shows that people eventually start to eat healthily on that seventh day and give up junk food entirely on their own accord, then I might get on board with this approach. But for now, I have other doubts as well.

A second problem with cheat days is that they encourage binge eating. If I know that I only have one day a week in which I can eat all the junk food that I have been deprived of for the last six days, what am I going to do? You got it—stuff my face with as much junk food and "comfort food" as I can. Forget that healthy stuff. So what if I add another one or two thousand calories to my weekly diet and lots of added fat, sugar, salt, and refined carbs just on that one day!

Finally, cheat days and cheat foods toy with the addictive centers of your brain. Junk food lights up those centers like a Christmas tree. Throwing gasoline on a fire you are trying to control is not going to make it easier to put that fire out. Rather, it only makes it that much harder not to eat junk food again the next day. Just ask anyone who has a non-food addiction if giving in to their addiction once a week helps.

If you adopt this or a similar diet, don't make them your final resting place. Use them as temporary crutches while you build up your ability to run the rest of the distance to the real finish line. Your goal is *not* to achieve partial good health. Your goal is to achieve outstanding health.

Can you have type 2 diabetes and not even know it?

The news recently reported on a study that showed that 1 in 7 Americans currently have type 2 diabetes and 30 percent—almost one in three—don't even know they have it.

Type 2 diabetes is a serious metabolic disease. Potential long-term complications include, among other things, heart disease, kidney damage, eye damage, foot damage, blood vessel disease, and even Alzheimer's disease. Being overweight is well-known for being a primary risk factor for the disease.

Some of us know this disease upfront and personal, having family members who have suffered for years and/or died from complications brought on by the disease.

But what if you find out that you have type 2 diabetes? Are there alternatives to just treating and managing the *symptoms* for the rest of your life at the expense of your lifestyle? Can type 2 diabetes be reversed? There is some evidence that it can, at least for some people (see Dr. Michael Greger's short video, "Reversing Diabetes with Food," at nutritionfacts.org, and Dr. Joel Fuhrman's book, *The End of Diabetes*).

Perhaps Hippocrates was right after all when he said. "Let food be thy medicine."

WEEK 13

"You have long-term vision when it comes to your health!"

"Eating right is self-care, not deprivation"

This quote from page 28 of Dr. Joel Fuhrman's latest book, *Fast Food Genocide: How Processed Food Is Killing Us and What We Can Do About It*, helped me realize that this is the exact mindset that anyone who is striving to eat healthily must acquire. When you feel deprived that you cannot eat junk food, your motivation to eat better is damaged. On the other hand, when you think, "I'll pass on junk food because I respect my body, feed it only the best fuel, and safeguard it from foods that are toxic to it," you feel empowered and your resolve is strengthened.

You can only believe it is a sacrifice to give up unhealthy food if you are ignorant about how nutritionally bankrupt, toxic, and harmful it is to your body. After all, most people today do not think it is a sacrifice *not* to smoke cigarettes.

Anyone who reads the first one-hundred pages of Dr. Fuhrman's book, for example, will never look at junk food the same way again. He lays out one consequence of eating junk food after another and substantiates it with a lot of research. And the way it is typically cooked makes it even deadlier. In the last few chapters, he discusses the healthy foods we should be eating instead.

People treat junk food lightly, but they shouldn't. According to Dr. Fuhrman's book, for example, research has shown that junk food can permanently alter your genes—including the ones that get passed onto your children—and that it is critical that children eat healthily and avoid junk food while they are young to avoid getting cancer later in life.

If you are having a hard time *wanting* to give up junk food or *giving it up*, you should definitely read his book. If you are a parent, you should likewise read his book because what you feed your children will have a lifelong impact on their health. In my opinion, this book should be "required reading" for all those who are wanting to get to healthy.

Where is your "happy place"?

I love the fall in the mountains that surround me. The air is cool, clear, and crisp; the skies are deep blue; the sun arcs low across the sky, casting acute-angle shadows that makes the mountains stand out in stark three dimensions; and the mountainsides are covered in a symphony of reds, oranges, yellows, and light and dark greens. Hiking in such spectacular scenery is breathtaking. One of my happy places is sitting on a mountain peak or ridge looking down and across the vast open valleys, craggy mountain peaks, and glacier-carved lakes.

Of course, I have other happy places as well, such as when I am with my children and grandchildren having a good time together. We all have happy places we go to both physically and mentally. I find that going to one helps me when I am laying in the dentist's chair getting a root canal.

Another of my happy places used to be sitting on a comfortable recliner with a big bowl of ice cream, a plate of freshly baked chocolate chip cookies, and/or a large bowl of buttered popcorn. Just thinking about it can still make me drool.

But after I became educated on healthy eating, I knew that this happy place had to go. It was only with great difficulty that I finally put it to rest. After all, junk food is addictive, self-soothing, fun to eat, and an easy emotional crutch. The problem is, it doesn't lead to good health. In fact, it's damaging to your health (see Dr. Joel Fuhrman's book, *Fast Food Genocide*).

So, review your list of happy places. If any of them include the scenario I just described, then perhaps it is time for a nutritional root canal—something that is painful to go through, but worth it in the end.

What kind of diet do your kids really eat?

Sometimes because we are so busy, we don't pay attention to what our kids are eating. We put food on the table, but do not check to see what our children actually eat. We buy crackers, cookies, cheese, yogurt, bagels, and chips for our pantries and refrigerators, and then turn a blind eye when our kids snack on them after school or during the evening when we are busy or out of the room. We send our kids off to play at their friends' houses, but don't think about what they might be eating while they are there. We give our kids lunch money, but don't follow up to ask what they ate for school lunch that day.

If this sounds like you, then you don't really know what kind of diet your kids are eating, and it is probably much worse than you think. For example, your kids might be eating 50, 100, or even 200 grams or more of added sugar in their diet every day without your even being aware of it.

The only way you can know this for sure is to put on your white lab coat and make a few careful observations. When you do, though, try to avoid relying on self-reporting, which is subject to significant bias because kids hide telling their parents about eating foods they know their parents will disapprove. Self-reporting, however, may be the only technique you have to find out what they ate at school or at a friend's house.

Direct observation, which is far superior, is best done without your kids knowing that you are observing them. People tend to change their behavior when they know they are being observed. Because it is difficult to observe and record food intake on more than one child at a time, just observe one of your children for a few days and then switch to another.

You might be surprised by what you learn. Kids are very skillful at being "picky eaters," selecting only those foods that have the most sugar, salt, fat, and taste appeal while avoiding more healthy alternatives. They also tend to "fill up" on unhealthy foods. You might even learn that one or more of your children is, for all intents and purposes, addicted to sugar and junk food, as manifested by their seeking out and eating only sugary or unhealthy foods.

Why does this matter? Because your children's futures depend on their eating a healthy diet. If kids go from meal to meal and snack to snack eating only junk foods and highly processed foods that are devoid of anything except calories, they are likely destined to live a shorter life and have serious health problems, starting in just a few short years.

Most kids eat massive amounts of raw calories from fast foods and junk foods, but very few micronutrients. Micronutrients are the antioxidants, fiber, and hundreds of phytonutrients that are found *only* in whole, plant-based foods. Micronutrients enable and facilitate proper cell functioning, extinguish cellular oxidative stresses, and help nullify the effects of toxic cellular waste products caused by normal cell metabolism which wreak havoc in our bodies over time if they are not neutralized or destroyed. Micronutrients are important to brain function, disease avoidance, IQ, longevity, the avoidance of depression, and overall vitality.

So, don't turn a blind eye to what your kids are eating. If they are eating mostly fast foods, junk foods, and highly processed foods, with very few—or little variety of—whole, plant-based foods, then a deafening five-alarm bell ought to be sounding in your head.

Likewise, don't take the easy road to feeding your kids, giving them largely what *they* want or what is cheap, easy, fast, and convenient. As a parent, your responsibility is *not* just to extinguish your children's hunger. It is to *deeply nourish* your children's bodies so that that they can have the brightest future possible and avoid unnecessary pain, suffering, disease, and diminished lives. If we love our children, don't we owe them at least that much?

Make it easy for your loved ones to eat healthily

Wouldn't it be nice if all we had to tell our kids at mealtimes is "go find some healthy food to eat in the refrigerator?" How many kids would follow through on tossing mixed salad greens or washing and cutting up fresh fruits and vegetables? How many would even microwave a bowl of frozen blueberries or peas to eat? How many would even know what healthy foods are?

In my experience, kids eat what is easy to eat—either things from a box or carton (processed foods), or food that is ready to eat that someone else has set in front of them. The challenge for parents, then, is to make it easy for your kids to eat *healthy* foods.

How is this done? By preparing healthy snacks, by putting a healthy meal on the table at mealtimes, by ridding your house of all unhealthy junk food, and by encouraging your kids to eat the healthy foods you give them. Most kids will eat at least some healthy food that is placed in front of them if they are encouraged to do so. And the more often they eat healthy food, the more likely they will accept it the next time and maybe even start liking it.

Fruits and vegetables are the most nutrient dense food on the planet. Prepare and set out some finger veggies such as grape tomatoes; sliced cucumbers; sliced red, yellow, and orange peppers; carrots; and celery (perhaps with some hummus for dipping). Place some fresh fruits and berries on your table that are washed, cut up, and ready to eat for dessert (just make sure they eat their other food first!). Put out some raw, unsalted nuts, another easy finger food that everyone should be eating every day. Serve side dishes containing whole grains and cooked vegetables. Prepare healthy snacks in advance and package them into small, individual storage containers that are ready to take out and consume.

My grandkids love things like oatmeal with raisins and cinnamon, homemade 100 percent whole wheat bread (made without oil), and fruit smoothies made with almond or soy milk (throw in a handful of fresh baby spinach into the blender when you make them).

It has been said that big things in life often turn on the seemingly small decisions that we make. It may seem like an inconsequential decision not to prepare and place a plate of fresh vegetables and fruit on the table along with other healthy, ready-to-eat foods, but over time, by so doing, you are severely stacking the odds against the health of your children and your family. Caring for others always carries the price tag of making sacrifices in time and effort for them. Let's do this for our children.

Farsightedness may be the key to long-term health

My eyesight has always been nearsighted, meaning I can only see things in-focus up close. I must wear corrective lenses to see things clearly that are far away so I can drive a car without running over a pedestrian or ski down a mountainside without colliding into a tree.

Are some of us nearsighted when it comes to our health, only worrying about it when we are sick or in pain? If so, then we need to put on the corrective lenses offered by researchers, doctors, and nutrition advocates who can teach us the long-term consequences of healthy and unhealthy eating. We want to see the red-flashing railroad sign or the sheer cliffs that are below us before it is too late.

Your ability to be farsighted is key to your long-term health. If you cannot see past your immediate dietary decisions (or if you are not even conscious of them) to see their long-term consequences, then you will eat like an American and you will die like an American (sounds patriotic, doesn't it). Unfortunately, many Americans will be dying prematurely—the upcoming generation is the first predicted to have a shorter lifespan than their predecessors, and they will die from diseases that could largely have been avoided through diet. Not only are we eating ourselves into an early grave, we are eating ourselves into a life full of unnecessary disease, pain, suffering, and expense.

Why is being farsighted so difficult when it comes to our health? Isn't this what we do in other aspects of our lives? We go to college or trade school so we can have a brighter economic future. We save up for a down payment on a house so we can purchase part of the American Dream. We put money aside into our retirement account every month so we can retire someday. We invest in our children's development and education so they will have a greater chance of success in life. We care for and nurture our relationships so that they will thrive and endure. All of these things are done with the long-term results in mind.

As Stephen R. Covey has said, we must "begin with the end in mind." We must choose our destiny and then align our lives to reach that end.

Now is the time for you to choose *your* health destiny.

More parents are taking their kids to fast-food restaurants

As reported recently by the news, a survey of 800 parents in the U.S. in 2016 showed that 91 percent said that they bought lunch or dinner for their child in the past week at one of the four largest fast-food chains in the country. I wonder how much closer this percentage would be to 100 percent if the researchers had included *any* fast food restaurant. Unfortunately, they did not mention if parents and their children went *more* than one time in the past week!

This is an increase of 79 percent from 2010. The reason for the increase, according to researchers, is that fast food restaurants have added more "healthy" options to their menus. Apparently, the strategy by marketers of offering a few "healthy" menu options is working—parents *feel good* about taking their kids to eat at a place that offers *some* healthy foods. However, once parents and their kids pass through the restaurant's doors, those healthy options are largely ignored. Kids (and their parents) are still largely ordering fast foods, not the "healthy" menu items.

The news article also mentioned that other research has shown that eating fast foods is associated with obesity, type 2 diabetes, heart disease and early death.

I hope such news is waking parents up to the reality that they are damaging their kid's health when they feed them junk food. Many parents seem to want to believe an alternate reality that because fast foods make their kids happy and satisfy their hunger, they must be good. Some parents also falsely believe that there is safety in running with the herd—and these herds are definitely feeding in fast-food pastures. Those who believe these false realities will have a rude awakening when the laws of nature catch up with them and their children.

Sadly, going out for fast food has become such an ingrained part of the American culture that it has probably surpassed baseball and apple pie as icons of our way of life. This means it is up to us as parents to change the eating culture we pass on to our children by making wise dining decisions.

Another fast-food brand gets a makeover

A national donut chain is the latest brand to get a new makeover, I believe because the public is starting to wise up as to how unhealthy donuts are in general. The company just announced that they are dropping the word "Donuts" from the name of their brand. Marketers are sensitive to changing public sentiment, so when one name falls out of favor, they simply rename the franchise or the product with a brand new one.

Some diet soda companies replaced the word "diet" with "zero sugar" in their product names. A major fried chicken restaurant dropped the word "fried" in their name by changing the name of its restaurants to three innocuous initials. Funny thing, though—it's all basically the same product as before, or one that is similar to the original. Once again, it's all about getting people to feel good again about buying their products. In marketing, it's all about the *feeling*, not the *reality*. Don't underestimate the power of marketing to persuade you to eat foods or drink beverages that might not do your health any favors.

WEEK 14

"You're definitely not a quitter!"

Should you eat plants or jellyfish to keep your brain healthy?

A television advertisement for a popular "brain health" supplement boasts how it contains an ingredient originally found in jellyfish. Sounds exotic, doesn't it (something marketers love)? But did Mother Nature really intend for us to eat jellyfish to keep our brains healthy? In centuries past and today, we don't all live by the sea, and even if we did, I don't think many people in centuries past ate poisonous jellyfish.

The news recently reported that 1 in every 2 women will get some kind of brain disease in their lifetime (such as dementia, Alzheimer's, or a stroke) and 1 in every 3 men. Those are pretty bad odds. So, what to do? Eat expensive jellyfish extracts?

No, it's much simpler than that. All we have to do is to eat a whole-food, plant-based diet that provides the hundreds of micronutrients and the healthy omega-3 oils (and their precursors) that we need for optimal health. It's no exaggeration to say that eating a whole-food, plant-based diet that also excludes all unhealthy foods is the most powerful deterrent to the leading causes of death from disease that afflict us today, including common brain diseases, such as stroke.

Dr. Joel Fuhrman's latest book, *Fast Food Genocide*, has over 90 pages referenced in the index under the entry "brain." His book documents that those who eat a whole-food, plant-based diet have better brain health, less brain fog, less brain disease, greater mental acuity and intelligence, better mood and emotions, and less depression than those who eat the standard American diet.

Additionally, Dr. Fuhrman shows how fast food, junk food, and processed foods actually damage our brains. He devotes an entire chapter to "The Brain on Fast Food." Our brains, as resilient as they are, cannot handle the continual and unchecked buildup of free radicals, other metabolic wastes, and toxic substances that come from eating such food. Many of these toxic and damaging substances are removed or nullified if we avoid eating junk food and eat enough phytonutrient-rich and antioxidant-rich foods our diet.

Be aware, though, that chemically extracting these micronutrients in little pills does not seem to be effective. They must be eaten in their natural form—in the whole, plant-based foods in which they are found—including green vegetables, seeds, berries, other fruits, mushrooms, nuts, beans, and whole grains.

So, eat your "phytos" everyday—not jellyfish—not just for your brain, but for your entire body. After knowing what you now know, you should never look at eating dark, leafy greens and other foods rich in phytonutrients and antioxidants the same again.

Is it good to eat like a king?

In centuries past, only royalty had access to and could afford to eat the fine meats and the fat-, sugar-, and calorie-laden foods that were placed on their massive dining tables. Today, we can all eat like kings. But is that a good thing?

I remember taking my grandchildren to a popular, all-you-can-eat local buffet that offered a huge selection of meats, white rolls and breads, salads, entrees, side dishes, soft drinks, and desserts. After we ate what seemed like two or three times the capacity of our stomachs, I would exclaim, "We ate like a king."

Unfortunately, eating like a king is not the royal road to a healthy life. In addition to the many diseases that we know come from eating this way, one illness—gout—was well-known to the people living in kingly times for afflicting royalty, cursing King Henry VIII and others.

Gout is extremely painful and is caused by needle-sharp crystals of uric acid that form in your joints. The formation of this acid is believed to be caused by alcohol consumption and by eating foods that are high in purines that break down in the body into uric acid. One food that is high in purines is meat. Although some plants also contain purines, eating plants does not appear to increase your chances for getting gout like eating meat and drinking alcohol do. In fact, they appear to be protective.

For more information, see Dr. Michael Greger's article "Plant vs. Animal Food Purines for Preventing Gout" on his website at nutritionfacts.org.

Food that is not food.

According to one news article, the Eskimos have over 50 words for snow. That got me thinking, maybe we need an equal number of words for food. After all, there is real food—fruits, vegetables, whole grains, legumes, nuts, mushrooms, and seeds—and then there are an endless variety of "fake" foods—foods that masquerade as real food. These include candy, chips, soda, fast food, ice cream, cake, cookies, pies, donuts and other bakery goods, cooking oils, and highly processed packaged and boxed foods that have altered ingredients and are full of white flour, sugar, salt, fat, and chemical preservatives and additives, perhaps with a few vitamins sprinkled back in (as required by law).

Maybe we should classify fake foods by the diseases they cause, by their level of nutritional deficiency, or by their minimum "safe" levels of daily consumption as determined by some third-party agency. On a more serious note, maybe we should put warning labels on fast food like we did with cigarettes.

Dr. Joel Fuhrman coined the term "Frankenfoods" to describe any fake food (such as fast foods, junk foods, and processed foods) that masquerades as real food. That seems perfectly descriptive to me, and it provides the necessary emotional overtones that should accompany fake foods. When someone asks you if you want to stop by a fast food joint for pizza or burgers, perhaps you should say, "No, thank you. I don't eat Frankenfoods." Maybe this response will get them to consider what they are about to eat!

Lumping both healthy and unhealthy foods under the same umbrella makes us feel better about eating Frankenfoods because we are, after all, "feeding" our bodies—a biological necessity. Food is food, right? We don't have to question the matter any further or think about what this particular "food" might be doing to our bodies.

Unfortunately, reality makes much finer judgments. All food is not food. Science tells us that some "foods" not only fail to provide our bodies with the deep nutrition they need, they actually harm our bodies, especially when they are consumed regularly.

So, the next time someone offers you fake food, just say, "I'll pass." Then go home and hang up a plaque in a prominent place where your whole family can see it that says, "Just say no to Frankenfoods."

Does dieting lead to permanent weight loss?

These days, diets are all the rage. An estimated 45 million Americans go on diets every year. Almost half of all Americans reported trying to lose weight between 2013 and 2016.

One of the latest fads in dieting is fasting. While research shows that continuous severe calorie restriction in mice leads to a longer lifespan, I have not heard of any similar studies done on humans, for obvious reasons!

Some people try to lose weight by skipping meals, especially breakfast. Some of the problems with this approach are a lack of energy throughout the morning and the tendency of people to overindulge at lunch due to excessive pent-up hunger and the "calorie credit" they feel they earned by skipping breakfast.

What about quick-weight-loss schemes? Do they work? Yes, some individuals have figured out how to manipulate the body in one unusual way or another to get rapid weight loss, and the faster the weight loss, the more popular the diet. But many of these unnatural diets are harmful to your body and should be avoided.

One diet, for example, emphasizes high protein and fat (from things like meat, eggs, butter, cream, cheese, and fatty fish) and low carbohydrates. Nutritionally, these are some of the worst foods you can eat. Processed meat, such as bacon and luncheon meats, and red meat, have been classified by the World Health Organization as Group 1 and Group 2 carcinogens, respectively. Meat (including fish), dairy, and eggs are full of saturated fat that is linked to cardiovascular and other diseases. Eating excessive protein overloads and stresses your kidneys. And, according to a recent news report, eating a diet that is too low in unrefined carbohydrates is harmful to your health.

When you learn about a new diet, the question you should ask yourself, after checking to see if the prescribed foods are healthy, is "What happens when people go off the diet? Do they regain the weight they lost six months or a year later?" According to scientific studies, 85 percent of dieters regain the weight they lost while dieting. Yo-yo dieting is more harmful to your health than if you never dieted (see Dr. Joel Fuhrman's book, *The End of Dieting*). And if people cannot sustain the "extreme" ways of eating (or not eating) required by a diet over the long haul, then what did the diet really accomplish, other than erode the person's self-esteem and possibly harm his or her health?

Consider this: Is it better for a roadside diner that follows unsanitary food preparation methods to spray for cockroaches every week or to change to more hygienic food practices? Similarly, do you want a quick dietary fix that does not last and may damage your health, or do you want a long-term weight-loss solution?

What Americans need today is not another diet. What they need is to change what they eat. When people eat a 100 percent whole-food, plant-based diet, they naturally shed excess weight, even without calorie restriction, and they keep that weight off as long as they continue to eat only healthy foods and refrain from eating fast food, junk food, cooking oils, processed foods, foods with added sugar, dairy—including cheese, milk, yogurt, and ice cream—and highly refined carbohydrates. And if they want to accelerate their weight-loss, they can just eat a few hundred less calories a day and bump up their exercise.

In short, eating a nutritarian diet—which is not a short-term "diet" but a way of eating that you stay on for the rest of your life—and slightly restricting your calories while getting adequate exercise is the best and most sustainable way to lose weight while still providing your body with optimal nutrition. The only side effect, besides the better health you will enjoy, will be the new wardrobe you will have to buy because of all the pounds you will permanently lose.

What you don't know about micronutrients can kill you

Our bodies need two kinds of nutrients to be healthy and function properly—macronutrients and micronutrients. *Macronutrients* are protein, fats, carbohydrates, and water. They provide the calories, water, and amino acids we need to burn energy and build tissues. Most diets focus on macronutrients, as did my public school education on nutrition. Food marketers love it when we focus on macronutrients because these are the very things they can easily manipulate in their processed foods and then boast about in their marketing messages.

Micronutrients are chemical elements or substances that are required for normal growth, development, cellular functioning, cellular repair, and the prevention of disease. Micronutrients include vitamins, minerals, antioxidants, and phytochemicals or phytonutrients ("phyto" means "plant").

While most people are aware that vitamins and minerals are necessary for good health, many have never heard of "phytonutrients" nor do they understand just how critical they are to our health, immune system, and disease resistance. Phytonutrients and antioxidants enable and facilitate proper cell functioning, extinguish oxidative stresses, help prevent cancer and other diseases, protect DNA, and help nullify the damaging effects of toxic cellular waste. They have a profound effect on human cellular function and on our immune system.

Micronutrients are so important that Dr. Joel Fuhrman defines the nutrient density of a food as the ratio of micronutrients in the food to calories (see page 180 in *Fast Food Genocide*). Remember, calories come from macronutrients (the denominator), so to increase the nutrient density, you have to increase the numerator—the micronutrients. The more micronutrients per calorie, the greater the nutrient density. By this definition, vegetables and fruits have the highest nutrient density of any food.

Micronutrients are so important to achieving excellent health and avoiding disease and early death that Dr. Fuhrman equates overall health with eating a sufficient amount and variety of nutrient-dense foods. He says that $H = N/C$. Health equals eating a diet of highly nutrient-dense foods.

How can you be assured that you are eating enough nutrient-dense foods and thereby getting sufficient antioxidants and phytonutrients in your diet? By following Dr. Fuhrman's nutritarian diet. When you eat the whole, plant-based foods prescribed by this diet, you will not only flood your diet with micronutrients (with the exception of vitamin B-12, which, if you don't eat meat, can be easily supplemented), you will automatically get adequate amounts of macronutrients, soluble and insoluble fiber, resistive and slowly digestible starches, and other health-promoting substances. In other words, you will likely be eating the healthiest diet on the planet.

While there are only two or three dozen vitamins and minerals, there are literally tens of thousands of phytonutrients, many of which have not yet even been identified. These are not substances that are found in the supplement aisle of your local health food store. In fact, the few that are in pill form have largely proven to be ineffective when they are extracted and isolated. Rather, they are only active and available in whole plant foods, such as colorful fruits and vegetables (including dark leafy greens), garlic, onions, whole grains, nuts, seeds, and legumes (beans, peas, chickpeas, and lentils). And yes, some are even found in *dark* chocolate (which is made from the cocoa bean).

Most importantly, phytonutrients are not found in animal products (meat, dairy, or eggs), which is a mainstay in the American diet, crowding out the eating of more nutrient-dense plant-based foods. Even the government erroneously treats meat as its own major food group in their nutritional pyramids. It isn't. Animal protein and animal fat have been linked to numerous serious diseases and health problems.

So, where are micronutrients found? In the produce section, in the frozen vegetable freezers, and in the bins selling whole grains, seeds, and raw nuts of your local grocery store.

Take a pizza, doughnut, or burger break

Ads appear all the time telling you that you *deserve* some product, service, or special privilege or that you should indulge yourself in their product because "you're worth it." Who does not remember a major fast food restaurant's wildly successful marketing song and tag line about our deserving a break today or the many ads for cosmetics and hair products that pitched "You're worth it"?

This is a powerful marketing tactic. When someone tells you that you deserve this or that, you start to wonder, "Maybe they're right." The real magic happens when you start to believe their flattery. That's when mental barriers to buying their product or believing their pitch start to come down.

Marketers continue to employ this same technique today. I recently saw an ad on TV for a candy bar that portrayed a busy person at work and touted, "You deserve a break"—a break, of course, to eat their product, which is exactly what they showed the person doing.

As a healthy eating advocate, what I want you to do is not to take a break to eat pizza, doughnuts, or a burger. What I want you to do is take a break *from* eating pizza, doughnuts, or a burger.

To that end, the next time you're thinking of eating out at a fast food restaurant, stay home and eat something healthy instead. Then, take the money that you would have spent on eating out and use it to purchase Dr. Joel Fuhrman's book, *Fast Food Genocide* or Dr. Michael Greger's book, *How Not to Die*. Either of these books cost less than a few bucks online. This onetime fast from eating out might forever change your life—if you follow through and read the book.

Having written and published four substantial books myself, I know just how many thousands of hours of labor it takes to write a serious book—especially one that collects, synthesizes, and distills scientific research from hundreds of sources, as Dr. Fuhrman's and Dr. Greger's books do.

Whether you realize it or not, we live in a time of real bargains when it comes to access to knowledge. When else in history could you tap into a lifetime of wisdom, experience, research, and knowledge from a perfect stranger for the cost of a modest meal? Remember, before the advent of books, only a handful of privileged people were allowed to sit at the feet of the wise to acquire such knowledge. Now, anyone can do so for less than an hour's wages. What an amazing opportunity! So, invest in your nutrition education. It will have far-reaching implications for you, your spouse, your children, and your posterity.

So, take a break today from your normal eating-out routine and buy the book. You're worth it!

A recipe for stuffed candy corn pizza—are you kidding?

One major processed-food manufacturer of frozen roll dough has figured out a new way to sell their product during Halloween season—by promoting a recipe on their website for stuffed candy corn pizza. This recipe doesn't really include candy corn as one of the ingredients (yes, another marketing tactic—bait and switch), but after you review the individual ingredients that follow, you will see that there are plenty of questionable ingredients to go around.

This recipe calls for 16 frozen dinner rolls, several cups of cooked chicken, 1 cup frozen corn, ½ teaspoon cumin, ¼ cup BBQ sauce, a jar of salsa con queso, 2 cups of shredded cheese, 2 cups of crushed nacho-flavored corn chips, and 1 cup of sour cream. In other words, this recipe takes one processed food and loads it up with several other processed foods, thus multiplying its nasty kick to your health.

Here is the breakdown of the Frankenfood (to use Dr. Fuhrman's term) ingredients that you will be placing into your body, just from the processed foods alone (these lists are taken from manufacturers' websites):

- White frozen roll dough: unbleached enriched white flour (wheat flour, malted barley flour, niacin, ferrous sulfate or reduced iron, thiamin mononitrate, riboflavin, folic acid), water, yeast, granulated sugar, soybean oil, salt, malt, sodium stearoyl lactylate, yeast nutrients (calcium sulfate, ammonium chloride), ascorbic acid, and enzyme.
- BBQ sauce: sugar, tomato puree, vinegar, apple cider vinegar, molasses, water, modified food starch, salt, natural hickory smoke

flavor, dried onions, mustard flour, dried garlic, spice, paprika, and potassium sorbate.
- Salsa con queso: water, skim milk, Monterey jack cheese (milk, cheese cultures, salt, enzymes), vegetable oil, modified corn starch, diced tomatoes in tomato juice, jalapeno peppers, chili peppers, red bell peppers, maltodextrin, salt, cheddar cheese, natural flavors, sodium hexametaphosphate, monosodium glutamate, datem, sodium phosphate, spice, and Yellow 5 and Yellow 6 food colorings.
- Nacho flavored corn chips: corn, vegetable oil, maltodextrin, salt, cheddar cheese, whey, monosodium glutamate, buttermilk, Romano cheese, whey protein concentrate, onion powder, corn flour, natural and artificial flavor, dextrose, tomato powder, lactose, spices, artificial color (including Yellow 6, Yellow 5, and Red 40), lactic acid, citric acid, sugar, garlic powder, skim milk, red and green bell pepper powder, disodium inosinate, and disodium guanylate.

To these, add the chicken, cheese, and sour cream—animal products that are full of salt and saturated fat and are linked to numerous health issues.

The serving suggestion displayed in the accompanying photo on their website shows the pizza being served with real candy corn on the side. If you do this, then add in:

- Candy corn: sugar, corn syrup, confectioner's glaze, salt, dextrose, gelatin (a protein made from animal parts like hides and bones), sesame oil, artificial flavor, honey, yellow 6, yellow 5, and red 3.

Scan over these ingredients listings and see how many of them represent whole, plant-based foods. Aside from the frozen corn, a tiny bit of finely diced peppers and tomatoes, a few natural spices, and a pinch or two of powdered vegetables like garlic and onions, there aren't any. The rest are chemical additives, highly refined flours, animal products, preservatives, conditioners, and other substances with names most of us cannot even pronounce. This is an unhealthy concoction of flavored chemicals, "enriched" flours, highly refined oils, and animal products—not whole, plant-based food.

After all, how many micronutrients, such as antioxidants and phytonutrients, do you think this "pizza" has? Not many. The few it has come from the less-refined plant-based ingredients that are found in tiny proportions, including a few spices. The nutrient density of this recipe is therefore extremely low.

Add to this dish the other highly processed foods and snacks most families eat every day, and what's a body to do?

WEEK 15

"Has junk food lost its luster yet?"

Learning to sing

Does your heart sing when you see your children, spouse, or grandchildren eating healthy food? Mine does. Why? Because I know just how important filling up on "supreme-grade" fuel—whole grains, vegetables, fruits, beans and other legumes, nuts, seeds, and other whole, plant-based foods—is to:

- Living a life full of vitality, energy, emotional wellness, and intellectual vigor,
- Living free of unnecessary pain, disease, and suffering, and
- Maximizing one's potential and personal fulfillment.

More specifically, every time I see my loved ones eat something healthy, I know they are helping to avoid:

- Becoming overweight or obese, along with its accompanying slew of health risks and problems—a real danger in America today,
- Heart disease, cancer of all types (including breast, colon, and prostate), type 2 diabetes, fatty liver disease, kidney disease, stroke, dementia, diminished IQs, acne, and a whole host of other health issues and diseases that are diet related or have major dietary contributing factors,
- Constipation, hemorrhoids, and other bowel and digestive tract issues because of all the fiber, slowly digestible starches, and micronutrients in the food,
- Depression and anger control issues (as shown by recent research—see Dr. Joel Fuhrman's book, *Fast Food Genocide*),
- Damage to the DNA they pass on to their children (again, as shown by recent research—see Dr. Fuhrman's book),
- Difficulty focusing their attention at school and in their jobs (ditto),
- Wildly fluctuating energy (blood sugar) levels with its periods of couch-potato lethargy and "sugar" highs,
- A lifetime of being burdened with multiple health issues and prescription medications with their accompanying serious side-effects and their loss of personal freedom, enjoyment, and potential,

- Incurring diseases that result in years or a lifetime of untreatable chronic pain that cost them a bundle in out-of-pocket healthcare expenses,
- The possible loss of employment and ability to earn a living, just when they reach their prime of life when their own spouse and children are entirely dependent on them, and
- The emotional devastation that always accompanies serious health crises.

At the same time, every time I see my loved ones eat something healthy, I know they are helping to:

- Avoid unnecessary physical pain and suffering (this alone should make it all worth it),
- Strengthen their immune systems against the many serious threats to their health (and possibly their life) that are out in the world, including the periodic endemics and epidemics that spread across the country unchecked,
- Add extra years to their lifespan,
- Protect their intellects (what they need to function and make a living) so they can use and rely on their brains their entire lives,
- Bolster their emotional resilience and well-being and strengthen their resistance to developing depression,
- Safeguard the DNA they are passing on to their children and posterity,
- Protect their pocketbooks against huge, unnecessary out-of-pocket healthcare expenses,
- Guard future life opportunities by making sure they have the health to pursue them,
- Make it easier, faster, and more pleasant to go to the bathroom,
- Maintain a healthy waistline, and
- Acquire the self-respect, self-discipline, and positive decision-making that taking responsibility for their health teaches.

Because I want my loved ones to enjoy these precious gifts—gifts that cannot be had in any other way—I get very excited when I can place healthy foods, such as fresh fruits and berries, warm steel-cut oatmeal with raisins and cinnamon, fresh vegetables, dark leafy greens, raw nuts, and home-made 100 percent whole-wheat bread fresh out of the bread maker, on the table in front of them.

If your heart hasn't been singing lately, then maybe you need to take a few vocal lessons—lessons on why healthy eating is so important. Your heart will be singing in no time!

Do you worry about your health as much as you worry about your mortgage?

Maybe you should. The typical home mortgage has a 30-year payback schedule. If you buy a house, say, when you're 25 years old, that means your loan would not be free and clear until you are age 55. By then, if you are eating the standard American diet (SAD), which Dr. Joel Fuhrman also calls the "deadly American diet," your chances of getting a progressive or metabolic disease, such as heart disease, cancer, diabetes, or some other serious health problem, is pretty good compared to those who eat a whole-food, plant-based diet.

For example, in Dr. Fuhrman's book, *Fast Food Genocide*, he quotes studies that show that a person eating a nutritarian diet has at least a hundredfold less risk of developing heart disease than a person eating the standard American diet (see page 17). He also reports that those who eat unhealthy foods such as fried foods, fast food, and processed foods, have ten times or higher the risk of heart attack compared to someone who eats a reasonably healthy diet.

So, if you want to increase your chances of being around when you pay off your mortgage and enjoy pocketing that extra money, you can either take out a shorter mortgage, or change what you eat.

The dangers of "recreational" eating

Would you consider using an illegal "recreational" street drug, such as speed or heroin? Probably not. Then why would you consider using a legal recreational "drug" which has similar addictive properties as street drugs and that lights up the same pleasure and addiction centers of your brain? Apparently, that's what happens when you eat foods containing either refined carbohydrates or added sugar—namely, junk foods and other highly processed foods.

Why? When these foods enter your digestive tract, they are quickly digested into simple sugars (monosaccharides) such as glucose that pass directly into your bloodstream. This triggers a rush of dopamine—a driver of addiction in your brain—and spikes your fat storage hormones, such as insulin, which convert the excess blood sugar into fat on your body.

As if that weren't bad enough, when you eat foods that contain both fats and sugar (or the equivalent of sugar—highly refined carbs), such as ice cream, donuts, or French fries, the pleasure centers in your brain explode with an even larger display of fireworks than the two do on their own.

When a person abuses any substance, the brain reacts by *reducing* the number of dopamine receptors, which means a person must ingest *more* of the substance to get the same pleasure from it as before (see pages 23 and 24 in Dr. Joel Fuhrman's book, *Fast Food Genocide*). Eating junk food creates a vicious cycle of eating more of it to get the same pleasure from it as before. This leads to addictive behavior and obesity. Have you ever noticed that eating the second, third, and subsequent potato chips or bites of ice cream doesn't cause the same rush of pleasure as the very first one? And who can stop after just one chip or spoonful?

Addiction and obesity, with its associated health problems, are not the only dangers of "recreational" eating. There are many other well-documented health risks that skyrocket when you eat unhealthy food over time. One of the most shocking but least well-known is that they actually damage the brain (see page 23 in his book).

So, the next time you set your sight on a burger, fries, ice cream sundae, donut, or other "recreational" junk food and the pleasure centers of your brain start to light up in anticipation, engage your frontal cortex of your brain and visualize what this food really is—a highly addictive and harmful substance that you would never consider taking.

Another fast-food restaurant announces a customer loyalty program

Another restaurant chain announced that it will be implementing a customer loyalty program to reward customers with points toward free food every time they make a purchase. Loyalty programs have been hugely successful—they attract new customers, increase sales, and bring past customers back into stores.

Before I made the change to healthy eating, I always made sure my loyalty card was punched every time I visited the local ice cream store. I couldn't wait to get that tenth punch so I could enjoy a free ice cream.

But is that what we need—another marketing strategy to entice people to eat more unhealthy junk food that damages their health? Probably not. But as long as we have a free society, people are free to make their own choices. Unfortunately, many people are making their choices in ignorance of the harm the "food" they are putting into their bodies will do to them.

Perhaps what we really need is an "infrequent eaters club" that rewards us for staying away from fast food and processed foods.

Junk food under the nutritional microscope

What happens when we put junk foods and other highly processed foods under the nutritional microscope? We find foods that are largely made up of macronutrients: carbohydrates, protein, and fat. The micronutrients—vitamins, minerals, antioxidants, and phytonutrients that are essential for health, cellular growth and repair, and disease prevention—are severely lacking. They were stripped out of the wheat kernels or rice kernels when they were processed.

Worse, junk foods and highly processed foods almost always come packaged with added sugar, salt, fat, preservatives, additives, chemicals, and toxins that are harmful or even carcinogenic (see Dr. Fuhrman's book, *Fast Food Genocide*, for a full and well-documented discussion of this topic). Did you really believe that the fine powder that comes out of a cake mix box is somehow nutritious?

To make matters even worse, food served at fast-food restaurants is typically fried or grilled, which greatly multiplies its toxicity and carcinogenic qualities.

Sadly, many Americans eat fast foods, junk foods, or highly processed foods at almost every meal, leading to what Dr. Fuhrman calls "excess-calorie malnutrition" with its accompanying chronic diseases and diminished lifespan and quality of life. As Dr. Fuhrman says, eating these kinds of food will literally kill you from the inside out in an act of "slow suicide."

Now that you know the rest of the nutritional story, what are *you* going to do?

Can you outrun your fork?

Many people believe that the best way to remedy America's trend toward obesity is to get people off their couches and into the gym. We are told that we are too lazy and that we need to discipline ourselves to "exercise off" our excess weight.

While regular exercise is an essential part of a healthy lifestyle, we are not going to exercise our way out of the current obesity crisis, at least according to leading health authorities. Why? Because exercise cannot compensate for the addicting and calorically dense fast foods, junk foods, and highly processed foods that we are eating.

In our country today, we eat mostly foods that were created by or processed in a factory or fast food restaurant—not foods taken directly from a farmer's field and placed on our tables unaltered. These artificially created foods are often loaded with highly refined carbohydrates (refined flours and added sugars), liquid and solid fats, and salt. In addition, we eat a lot of meat, which is riddled with fat and other unhealthful things.

On the other hand, natural, whole foods are the kind that grow out of the ground or on a tree. They are full of fiber, water, and non-digestible and resistant starches that quickly fill up your stomach and cause your stretch sensors to tell your brain to stop eating.

Processed foods lack any significant amounts of fiber, so your brain is not notified that you are full. They digest quickly, dumping excess sugar and fat into your bloodstream, which are quickly stored on your body as fat. Moreover, they are addictive, which leads to further calorie intake.

If we are serious about tackling today's obesity crisis, we must change what we eat—not how much we eat or even how much additional exercise we must do. When we eat the foods that nature designed for the human body, we get just the right amount of calories we need to sustain a healthy weight while feeling full and satisfied—and we provide our bodies with optimal nutrition.

So, while you cannot outrun your fork, you can change *what* you pick up with your fork—and that makes all the difference in the world.

Have car, will travel—and eat!

This summer, my wife and I drove to Bryce Canyon National Park, where we hiked extensively for three days. We didn't eat out once, knowing that there would be few or no healthy choices at the two or three local eateries in this remote location. Instead, we purchased a couple of long coolers on wheels with slide-out handles and took all our food with us.

The large bag of ice that I put in each cooler lasted for the three days. We only had to add a little more from the hotel ice machine at night. We used the microwave oven in the hotel room to heat and cook our food and ate on paper plates to avoid doing dishes. We didn't miss a beat as far as our diet was concerned—we just ate the food we usually do. All that was required was a little advanced planning and packing.

WEEK 16

"Doesn't it feel good to take your health destiny into your own hands?"

"Who cares if I die a few years earlier?"

Some people don't worry about eating healthily because they tell themselves that they would rather eat all the pizza, burgers, fries, ice cream, chips, candy, cakes, cookies, donuts, and commercialized foods that they want and die a few years younger than be "miserable" all those years from abstaining from "pleasure foods." While on some level this may sound like a reasonable proposition, it doesn't tell the whole truth.

While it is true that you will likely die far sooner by eating an unhealthy diet, death is not your only worry. Your body is an amazing creation. *It doesn't want to die.* It will try to hang in there and stay alive through all kinds of nutritional abuse, threats, and diseases for as long as it can. However, it does not do so without a price. Part of that price (beside the financial cost) is the physical pain, loss of normal bodily function, and the limitations in personal freedom and capability that result from impaired health.

Physical pain from health problems comes from two sources. First is the pain that is caused directly by the disease itself and is one of its symptoms. This pain in-and-of-itself can be excruciating. Second is the physical pain caused by the medical procedures, interventions, and treatments you undertake for the disease.

In the latter category are things like surgery, biopsies, invasive procedures (such as cardiac by-passes and stents), tests of all kinds, cancer treatments—including radiation and chemotherapy—and the nasty side-effects of pharmaceutical medications (as one physician rightly said about what his instructor told him in medical school, "all medications have side-effects"). Those who have insulated themselves from the truly ill have little comprehension of just how intense this pain can be and how difficult it can be to endure. Indeed, death is sometimes seen by those suffering from chronic pain as a welcome relief.

Some have said that we live in a time of medical delusion in which we put highly skilled and intelligent doctors, pharmaceutical companies, and high-tech medical equipment providers on pedestals, treating them like gods and believing that they have in their back pocket a quick cure for almost anything that might afflict us. However, those who have experienced serious health issues themselves and those who are close to others who suffer know just how far from the truth this delusion is.

Yes, medical procedures, medicines, and devices can truly save lives and are godsends for certain medical conditions, diseases, and emergencies. But modern medicine is far from curing many common diseases such as cancer, heart disease, type 2 diabetes, and Alzheimer's, and is far from offering an effective, safe solution for chronic pain (consider the current opioid crisis). Meanwhile, human suffering from disease continues on an impressive scale and millions of lives are cut short or are left contracted and unrealized.

So, perhaps it is not dying or shaving off a few years that should be your big concern. After all, death is a certainty for everyone who is born into this world. Rather, your real concern should be how much you want to suffer, how intensely you want to suffer, and for how long you want to suffer *before* you die?

How one company encourages healthier eating on-the-job

A major high-tech company based in Mountain View, California, offers its employees free food day-or-night in its many on-campus cafeterias. To encourage healthier eating, it labels its food offerings with traffic-light colors: green means "eat anytime," yellow means "eat only once in a while," and red means "do not eat often." The prices of items in its vending machines, which are not free, are based on their nutrient content—healthy foods sell for less and unhealthy snacks sell for more. The ultimate goal of the company is to reduce healthcare costs by improving the health of its employees.

As progressive as these tactics may be, ultimately, it is best if you develop your own skill at assessing the health value of the food you are considering eating. One of the keys to making this assessment is to ignore all of the marketing hype on the front of the package and look directly at two things found elsewhere on the package: the *ingredients listing* and the *Nutrition Facts* table.

If the ingredients listing has added fat, oil, or sugar of any kind; white ("enriched") flour; meat, eggs, or dairy products; other highly processed ingredients; or names of chemicals, preservatives, colorings, or enhancers, then you should probably put it back.

Likewise, if the Nutrition Facts label has any of the following, then you should probably put it back:

- An unrealistic serving size that makes the numbers in the Nutrition Facts table look much better than they really are,
- More than 3 or 4 grams of sugar per serving (zero added sugar is best),
- A high percentage of overall fat (little or no fat is best, unless it is fat from whole foods containing healthy fat that were added to the product, such as nuts, seeds, or avocados),
- Anything but very little or no salt (sodium),
- Anything but zero cholesterol,
- Anything but zero trans-fat, or
- More than 5 times the number of grams of carbohydrates as the number of grams of fiber (for example, 30 grams of carbohydrates but only 5 grams of fiber is 6 times the number of grams of fiber, so put it back).

This is quite different than what some food advertisers tell us, which is to focus on the number of grams of protein a product has and ignore almost everything else. Nutrition bars, for example, typically brag about how much protein they have (much of which comes from added protein powders or refined protein sources) while ignoring all the added oil, fat, salt, and sugar they contain. What most people don't realize is if you eat a whole-food, plant-based diet (such as a nutritarian diet) you will automatically meet all of your protein needs without eating meat and without artificially trying to bump up your protein intake.

Likewise, when you go out to eat, avoid dishes and foods that are made with:

- Meat, eggs, and dairy products such as cheese, cream, yogurt, or ice cream,
- Refined flours (such as white breads and pasta),
- Added sugar,
- Added oils, or
- Any other highly refined ingredient.

What's left, you ask? Not much—usually just the fresh foods served at the salad bar, but only if you eat them without the prepared dressings, which are loaded with oil (100 percent fat). But this is the point—most restaurants do *not* serve healthy food—food that doesn't damage your health over the long haul (and possibly even over the short haul) and food that truly nourishes your body.

If you want to eat healthily, you will probably have to eat mostly at home from meals you have personally prepared. If you go on the road, your safest bet is to prepare healthy food in advance and take it with you. This takes more forethought and effort, but, as Dr. Joel Fuhrman says, "Good health cannot be bought—it must be earned."

Understanding your daily vulnerability cycle

When I wake up in the morning after a good night's sleep, I feel rejuvenated, healthy, and ready to jump into another day's activities. My body feels well-nourished from all the healthy food I ate the day before, and I have no trouble resisting any temptations to eat junk food. Unhealthy food just isn't attractive to me. Drive me by all the fast food restaurants you want or walk me through all the candy, chip, and ice cream aisles at the grocery store and I still won't be phased.

However, later in the evening, after the day's activities, challenges, and issues have made their significant mental, emotional, and physical withdrawals, the siren call to eat unhealthy food can sometimes be a real temptation. In the matter of a few hours, my brain has gone from seeing junk food for what it is to toying with the idea of eating it to boost my energy, sooth my frayed emotions, or just provide me some pleasure (addictive substances release dopamine in the brain). This is when the strong tentacles of the pleasure trap threaten to sneak up and engulf me.

If this has ever happened to you, then what can you do to address this problem? Here are a few tips. First of all, evening is not the time to eat a late dinner. If you have gone more than four or five hours since lunch, your brain is already tempting you to stop by after work for a hamburger, pizza, or a dozen donuts. Children are even more sensitive than adults to going without food because of their smaller stomachs; they typically need an intervening mid-afternoon snack. Eating on time addresses hunger pains before they intensify and get out-of-control and before your energy levels dip to uncomfortable levels, both of which trigger your brain to focus its attention on how to quickly resolve this "urgent" biological need.

Second, when you do eat, eat a healthy meal and eat until you are full. Eat a delicious nutritarian or vegan entrée (which can be leftovers from the previous day) full of satisfying spices, flavors, and textures—one that you like—so that you will feel like you just dined on some amazing gourmet food. Also eat a few whole foods that have healthy fats in them, such as a half an avocado, a palmful of nuts, or some nutritious seeds. The spices, natural sugars, and healthy fat in these foods will trigger the sensors in your stomach that detect the "richness" of your food and signal your brain that you are getting enough calories. Healthy fats, which are always accompanied by fiber, also extend the time it takes to digest your meal, keeping your energy levels more stable throughout the evening.

As part of your dinner, eat a generous portion of cooked and raw vegetables and some grains or legumes, such as brown rice, beans, peas, corn on the cob, cooked wheat kernels, or quinoa. This fills out your meal with plenty of fiber and triggers the stretch receptors in your stomach that you are full. Finally, satisfy your craving for sweets by eating some fresh or frozen fruits or berries, making a fruit smoothie, or eating a slice of watermelon or cantaloupe.

In short, your first line of defense is to eat on time, eat until you are full, and eat a healthy meal containing whole, plant-based foods.

Your second line of defense is to spend your after-dinner time in satisfying and fulfilling activities. Play ping pong, foosball, or a board game with your children or grandchildren. Go for a walk or to the park. Read an interesting book. Learn something new. Make or build something with your hands. Watch a good movie. Socialize with your friends. Play a musical instrument. Develop your talents. Write a book. Help others. When you are intellectually, emotionally, and socially engaged, you will be less likely to rely on junk food as an emotional crutch, to feel good, or to appease feelings of social isolation.

When junk-food cravings do occur, recognize them for what they are—built in, biological motivations to seek pleasure, avoid pain, and minimize effort—motivations that, in this case, will lead you to damaged health, expanded waistlines, and addiction to pleasurable but toxic foods. Intense cravings typically last only a few minutes, so distract yourself and remember that what feels right at the moment isn't necessarily good for you. Recognize that the longer you abstain from junk food, the less intense these cravings become and the less frequently they occur.

Next, avoid skipping breakfast or lunch, which catches up with you later in the day—even though you ate an intervening meal—and make sure these other two meals are healthy too. If your body is deprived of real nutrition, when evening arrives, your resolve is already compromised.

Finally, go to bed on time. Running a sleep deficit from day to day is Kryptonite to your powers of resistance. Studies show that you eat more when you are sleep deprived. Sleep deprivation is painful to your brain, and it will seek out ways to immediately stop the pain and replace it with something that is pleasurable.

Is healthy food bare, naked food?

At the store the other day, I passed a marketing display for natural, organic soaps. The caption at the top of the display read, "Any more natural and you'd be naked." It got me thinking, "Does this apply to healthy food?" I believe it does. Healthy food is bare, naked food.

Naked food is whole food in its natural, unaltered state—food that hasn't gone through machines or factories that transform it into something else, like a flour factory in which raw wheat kernels drop from hoppers at one end, nutrients are stripped out, and bags of white, bleached flour exit the other end. Naked food is recognizable for what it is. You can easily identify it just by looking at it. There is no deception, alteration, or transformation into an unnatural state by mechanical or chemical means.

If you could see the raw ingredients that make up the recipes for most processed foods—the bags of powders and vats of liquids that are the refined flours, additives, taste enhancers, conditioners, coloring agents, sugars, hydrolyzed fats, oils, chemicals, and preservatives—you would be unable to recognize any of those ingredients as real food. They have no recognizable identity. Many are not even extracted from real foods—they are artificially created by mechanical or chemical means. But people are fooled. They think that because the resulting "food" has calories, looks appealing in its new form, and tastes great, that it is "food" and is therefore okay to eat.

When you ponder a visualization of these raw ingredients, you should ask yourself, "How can my body even digest this toxic brew of micronutrient-stripped ingredients and artificial (and often toxic) chemicals?" The answer is, not very well, and not without impacting your waistline and your health, as evidenced by the spiraling trends in many serious and life-threatening diseases.

What about the food you prepare at home using bare, naked foods as ingredients? Don't they undergo a "transformation"? Yes they do, but the transformation is one that simply alters the *form* of the whole food—*not* the nutrition! Nothing has been stripped out or processed away. All of the original whole-food molecules—including the fiber and micronutrients—are all preserved in the final dish. The only thing that has changed is the shape or form of the ingredients when they were blended, mashed, chopped, combined, or cooked. The final dish is still just as nutritious as the original collection of whole foods.

So, before letting your senses fool you into thinking that the candy bar, loaf of white bread, or rehydrated macaroni and cheese looks and tastes good so it must be good, read the ingredients listing and visualize just what those ingredients looked like when they arrived at the factory. If they aren't bare, naked foods whose molecules were left unaltered, then put it back.

Still need more convincing? Then tour a processed food factory and see for yourself.

Your last defense

The national news recently aired a story about the rise of AFM (Acute Flaccid Myelitis). While this disease is very rare, it is afflicting an increasing number of children in the U.S. with polio-like symptoms and paralysis. While the cause of the disease is unknown at this time, the story made me think about future possible epidemics in which an illness or disease is communicable from person to person.

Because epidemics are often caused by new diseases or variants of existing diseases, there will likely be no vaccinations for them and very limited treatment options. This allows them to spread across the population unchecked. Sadly, children and the elderly are often the first to succumb, with death taking the defenseless across all socioeconomic boundaries.

When an epidemic like this hits, it will be too late to take a magic pill to protect yourself, your spouse, and your children and make the danger go away (where would you get such a pill anyway?). Your last defense will be your body's own immune system. If this defense is breached, then your chances of survival are dim. However, with a strong immune system, even if you do get infected, your chances of survival are much greater, and recovery times, if you do recover, will most likely be shorter than they would have been otherwise.

Of course, a strong immune system is useful for much more than just an occasional epidemic. It is your last defense for a variety of illnesses, parasites, microorganisms, and diseases that attack your body daily. Without it, a simple common cold would be deadly. Running on a weak immune system is like running an engine on only two cylinders—you have very little disease-fighting horsepower and you are more likely to break down or simply give up the ghost.

If you are eating the standard American diet, you are doing yourself double injury. Not only are you failing to provide the nourishment your body so desperately needs, you are damaging your cells, impeding bodily function, and promoting disease. This is what fast foods, junk foods, and highly processed foods do (see Dr. Joel Fuhrman's book, *Fast Food Genocide*). By eating the standard American diet, you are, in a very real sense, crippling part of your immune system.

So, start now to build up your immune system. Make your last defense be your best defense. Arm your body with the best possible weapon it can have—a strong immune system. Eat a whole-food, plant-based diet filled with a rich variety of fruits, vegetables, whole grains, legumes, cooked mushrooms, nuts, and seeds. This will deeply nourish all the cells and organs of your body so they can perform at their best and store up critical reserves of antioxidants, vitamins, minerals, and phytonutrients that can be called upon under stressful circumstances.

Another fast-food distribution channel extends its reach

It seems that the creativity of fast-food marketers is just about endless. Getting their unhealthy wares in front of you in non-traditional ways and locations has always been on their plate. Now it is getting yet another boost. My local TV news station recently announced that vending machines selling raw cookie dough are coming to my state—a move that was applauded and cheered by everyone in the newsroom.

As amazed as I was by this announcement (and the reaction of those in the newsroom), I was even more taken aback when I did an online search and found photos of dedicated vending machines selling pizza, cooked sausage, French fries, and mashed potatoes and gravy. Sadly, I'm sure that even these off-the-scale unhealthy foods sound tempting and delicious to many people.

I started to wonder how many of these machines will show up on college campuses, in hospital waiting rooms, in high school lunch rooms, at hotels, and in other public spaces such as airports, train stations, and bus stations? But on further reflection, maybe the proliferation of fast-food vending machines isn't the real problem. As much as I as a consumer might want to blame fast food vendors for our nation's diminishing health, the truth is, they are not the ones to blame. We are!

How so? Consider this: In a free marketplace, businesses offer goods and services that consumers are willing to buy. As consumer tastes, preferences, and trends change, business must also change or go out of business. That is how free enterprise works. The demand in the marketplace is what drives the goods and services that businesses offer, and we are the ones who define that demand every time we make a purchase. As proof of this assertion, have you ever wondered what would happen to the illegal drug business in our country if no one bought illegal drugs?

Take a moment to reflect on the implications of these simple facts. Then, ask yourself, "What is my contribution to our current food landscape? When I pull out my wallet at a grocery store, vending machine, or convenience store, am I supporting the marketing and selling of unhealthy junk food, or am I motivating businesses to stop selling junk and offer healthy foods?"

Can the culture you were born into kill you?

Humans exist as social creatures. We are born into a collective culture comprised of peoples, traditions, group identity, and nationality. Our culture is what is "normal" to us. It eludes our consciousness until it is superimposed on a different culture or we are immersed in another culture. It has a powerful influence on our beliefs, goals, and preferences—including our food preferences.

Our food culture consists of the foods we love, buy, and prepare, as well as our physical "food institutions"—the fast food restaurants, convenience stores, and supermarkets that can be found on almost every corner of suburbia. Most of us grew up frequenting these restaurants and eating these foods. Our individual and collective identify is strongly tied to them, and we typically never give them a second thought.

But maybe we should. What if our culture is supplying us with mostly unhealthy foods? What if our culture has molded our food preferences from a young age to prefer junk foods and processed foods that are dangerous or even toxic to our health (see Dr. Joel Fuhrman's book, *Fast Food Genocide*)? If so, then maybe it is time that we take action. After all, if an enemy state were insidiously invading our country and killing millions of people every year by poisoning our food or water supply, we wouldn't just sit passively by and do nothing.

Taking action will not be easy. Our culture has an iron grip on us. No one wants to be seen as a non-conformist or a cultural offender. When we go out to eat with our colleagues at work or go to a friend's house for dinner, we don't want to be seen as different, rude, or out-of-step with what is "normal." Everyone wants to fit in and feel the emotional satisfaction of being "part of the group." This desire for social unity is a powerful force that bind groups and societies together.

Changing our culture is very challenging. Marketers spend billions every year trying to do just that. Sometimes, culture change requires early adopters who are willing to set the example and to teach others by example a better way. These non-conformists, however, are often subject to intense scrutiny, public criticism, social ostracism, ridicule, and even persecution.

So, what can you do? Quietly change your own food culture and tactfully educate others on the benefits of healthy eating while respecting their freedom to choose. Remember, it took several decades for our culture to catch up with the science that showed that smoking caused cancer and heart disease. Meanwhile, millions needlessly suffered and perished. Don't be a victim of culture lag.

WEEK 17

"Have your taste buds made the switch yet?"

Let not thy tongue be thy guide

Several times a week, employees at a wholesale club that I frequent set up tasting tables where free food samples are handed out. Outspoken hucksters stand behind small tables where they use toaster ovens, griddles, electric pots, and microwaves to heat up samples of the store's frozen or refrigerated processed foods. During the days leading up to holidays, they often hand out ready-to-eat samples of junk foods such as cookies, candies, chips, or limited-time-offer novelty foods ("get them while you can").

These sampling stations are extremely popular and create shopping cart congestion all around them as adults and kids scramble to grab a sample from the offering trays before they quickly disappear. Someone must think these booths are a huge success because they show up repeatedly all year long.

I find it interesting to stand back and watch the reactions of the store patrons as they sample the food. Their first and biggest concern seems to be how the product tastes. Because almost all junk food triggers one or more of the pleasure centers of the brain, the product is usually a big hit. Customers smack their lips and exclaim "This really tastes good!" Only after verifying that the product tastes good do they check out the price. Because the foods selected for sampling are typically products that are new or not well known, these same customers are delighted to "discover" a new junk food to feed themselves and their family.

Unfortunately, I am one of the few people who pick up the display box and read the ingredients listing and Nutrition Table that is "hidden" on the back, side, or bottom of the package. This usually confirms my suspicions that the product contains several unhealthy ingredients and should not be eaten. Nevertheless, the availability of this information does not seem to deter the popularity of these items.

Could it be that our culture has trained us to have a single criterion by which we judge the food we put into our bodies? "If it tastes good, go for it!" Sadly, the nutritional value of the food and its potential to injure our health doesn't seem to enter into the equation. If it triggers the sweet, salt, and/or fat receptors on our tongues, then we give it two enthusiastic thumbs up without ever considering the product's health implications.

It has been said that the tongue is a little member of the body that has a huge potential for verbal mischief. Perhaps it is time that we recognize that the tongue is a little member of the body that has a huge potential for nutritional mischief.

Use your brain—not your taste buds—to evaluate whether you should eat a potential food.

Does how you eat affect our environment and our planet?

Here are a few sobering facts:

- The livestock sector contributes more carbon dioxide emissions than the entire world transportation sector (all of the cars and trucks combined).
- The 300 million tons of manure produced by factory farms in the U.S. account for 37 percent of agricultural greenhouse emissions.
- It takes many times more water to produce one pound of animal protein than one pound of grain protein
- 70% of the arable land in the U.S. is used to grow crops for animals and not humans, and worldwide, almost a third of arable land is used for animal agriculture
- The excrements of 80 billion land animals raised for food every year are left untreated and go back to our water basins and oceans, polluting our waters.
- Around 5 million acres of rainforest are destroyed every year by the livestock industry worldwide.

Eating plants is not only more sustainable, it is far better for the planet.

Watch out for all that extra food you eat at work

The news recently reported on a study that showed that workers eat almost an additional 1,300 calories of food and beverages per week in the workplace from vending machines, commons areas, meeting rooms, and worksite social events. This is more than half of the recommended daily calorie intake for the average adult!

Because you will gain 1 extra pound for every 3,500 additional calories you eat, you will add about a pound and a half a month onto your weight unless you cut down on eating other foods at mealtimes. But it wasn't just the raw calories. The foods at work tended to be high in salt and full of "empty" calories—foods like pizza, soft drinks, cookies, brownies, cakes, and candy. These foods dump a huge sugar load into your body as well. Maybe what we need are vending machines that dispense fresh vegetables, fruits, nuts, and seeds instead!

Just because something is socially acceptable, done in a group, or commonplace does not mean that it is good for you.

Another upcoming fast food trend

A major national newspaper reported that a major chicken sandwich fast food franchise is expanding into offering full meal kits on a trial basis at some of its Atlanta outlets. These are kits that customers can pick up at the drive-thru or front counter. They will offer five different entrees. Each kit will serve two people. They are designed to be prepared in your own home in about 30 minutes. The article mentioned that meal kits are growing in popularity and now generate more than $2 billion a year in revenue. It appears that fast food has invented yet another way for consumers to get their junk food fix.

Fast food outlets seem to cater to those who never want to have to plan a meal in advance or even think about what they are going to eat, other than choosing where to go out to eat. But when you plan and prepare your own healthy meal kits, you will never get caught needing to run to the local fast food store to buy three of their kits to serve your family of four kids and two adults—which, by the way, will set you back a wad of cash.

Although there may be prepared food providers that offer healthy meal kits where you live, why not make them yourself and save some money? I prepare my salads, soup, nuts, seeds, fresh veggies for munching, and fresh berries once a week and put them into containers that can simply be taken out of the fridge and eaten (or washed and eaten, in the case of berries and grapes). The healthy entrees I make will last for two or three days, so I don't have to cook every day.

I keep other ingredients such as quinoa, steel cut oats, brown rice, sweet potatoes, fresh fruits, nuts, whole-wheat bread, almond milk, and fresh and frozen fruits and vegetables, stocked and on hand so they can be quickly assembled and eaten. Aside from my food preparation days, my meal times typically take five to ten minutes to gather, warm up or cook, and serve. How's that for fast food!

Avoiding medical insurance nightmares

At the time you select a medical insurance plan, the insurance companies always put on their best face. Their message is reassuring, simple, and straightforward: "Pay only a certain co-pay or a certain percentage of the cost of the visit or procedure, perhaps after you reach your personal and family deductible, adjusted by whether the providers are 'in-network' or 'out-of-network.'"

The underlying message is, "We've got you covered." But in practice, the reality is far different and is often tangled up in a web of confusing special qualifications, restrictions, and hidden exceptions. The real details often have to be extracted out of the company over the telephone by lawyer-like cross-examinations with hard-to-understand call-center representatives. Even then, you are not always confident that you can trust their answers, which can vary across calls. The whole process can be a real nightmare and can take many hours or days to complete.

Just because your doctor refers you to a specialist or puts in an order for a procedure does not mean your bases are covered. Much more is required. The responsibility is on you to check at every point in the process to ensure that you are in absolute compliance with the insurance company's policies and procedures—or risk having to pay all of the costs yourself. No one else is going to do this for you.

Anyone who has used their insurance for a major medical procedure knows just how difficult it can be to make sense of the maze of procedures, inconsistent call-center statements, and uncertain coverages. Even duly authorized call-center agents often say that "What is actually covered in your specific case will be in accordance with what your several-hundred-page policy states that is secreted away somewhere in our corporate vault." "But," you thought, "isn't that why I called you the first place?"

Here are some of the things you will likely have to do:

- Find out if the procedure is "covered" by your insurance.
- Find out if the specialist you want to see is "in-network" and if they accept your particular insurance plan.
- Find out if the hospital or out-patient clinic (the facility itself) where the procedure will be performed is "in-network" and if so, verify independently that they accept your particular insurance plan.

- Find out the names of everyone who will be involved in the surgery or procedure, including the surgeon, the anesthesiologist, the surgical assistants, the x-ray or MRI technician, and the physician "reading" the x-rays or scans. Then find out if they accept your insurance. If so, call your insurance company and find out if each one is "in-network." As it turns out, providers can "accept" a particular insurance and still not be "in-network."
- Find out from your insurance company if the procedure requires advanced "pre-authorization." If so, ask your referring physician's office to secure a pre-authorization for the procedure from the insurance company. Then, follow up a few days later to make sure they really received it. Otherwise, you may be responsible for paying the entire cost of the procedure yourself, which could amount to thousands of dollars!
- Check your prescription and lab coverage. Then check to see if your pharmacy accepts your insurance. Check to make sure the laboratory doing your lab work is "in network."

If all this doesn't make your head spin and test the limits of your patience, then just wait until you get your medical bills from the physicians, technicians, assistants, laboratories, clinics, hospitals, and out-patient facilities that serviced you during your procedure or stay. The sticker shock from these bills alone may give you a heart attack! Look at each bill and try to figure out what the charges were for and how they were computed. Try to see which charges were already submitted to the insurance company, and if so, what your insurance paid and didn't pay. Studies reported on by a leading consumer magazine show that bills are often inaccurate. If so, you may have to "go to battle" with each provider's billing department and/or your insurance company.

Perhaps you have heard that those who are diagnosed with cancer fight two battles. One is the life-or-death battle against cancer. The other is the fight against their insurance company. Where are the consumer advocates and the consumer protections in all this?

The bottom line is this: How often do *you* want to subject yourself to this doubly painful experience? The answer is determined by your actions, not your desires. It depends on what you eat. If you eat like an American, you will visit the doctor, the surgeon, the specialist, the out-patient clinic, and the hospital as frequently as most Americans on average and enjoy this frustration far too often.

Instead, why not keep your visits to rare occasions by eating a whole-food, plant-based diet—one which has proven to build your immune system, prevent disease, and improve your health better than any other diet?

Salt—the other "white stuff"

Added sugar is not the only villain in our diets. Too much salt (sodium chloride, or NaCl) also damages our health. Most people have heard that excess salt raises blood pressure (actually, it turns out to be a linear relationship, not an inverted U-shaped relationship), but nevertheless think of salt as a fairly benign substance, shaking it generously on their French fries, meats, and other foods and adding it to their favorite recipes by the measuring spoonful.

Many people are unaware that the standard American diet (SAD), with its high amounts of fast foods, junk foods, and highly processed foods, is already overloaded with salt. Manufacturers and food processors (including producers of meat, poultry, and fish) add or inject salt to enhance flavor, increase appetite, increase thirst (fast food restaurants want you to buy more soda, one of their most profitable items), and entice you to come back for more.

Astonishingly, according to Dr. Michael Greger, 75 percent of all dietary salt comes from processed foods. The single greatest source of dietary salt for those between the ages of 20 and 50 is chicken, which has salt injected into the meat (see nutritionfacts.org).

According to Dr. Joel Fuhrman (see his book, *Fast Food Genocide*), added salt in your diet:

- Increases blood pressure, which stresses your heart and blood vessels and increases your risk of heart attack, heart failure, and stroke; in fact, according to Harvard's T. H. Chan School of Public Health, high blood pressure accounts for two-thirds of all strokes and half of all heart disease,
- Causes scarring of the heart (coronary fibrosis), which can lead to cardiac arrhythmia or irregular heartbeat,
- Increases your risk of developing asthma, autoimmune disease, stomach cancer, osteoporosis, and kidney failure,
- Interferes with your cues to stop eating when you are full (dieters, are you reading this!), and

- "Deadens" the salt receptors in your taste buds after repeated use, which encourages you to add even more salt to your food to maintain that "salty" taste.

You would think that with all of these known, serious consequences, we would stop viewing salt as a benign substance and instead view it as something to avoid.

Although a certain amount of sodium is essential to normal bodily functioning, eating a whole-food, plant-based diet that includes a wide variety of plant-based foods already provides a sufficient amount of natural salt that is still under the maximum limit of 1,500 mg a day that is recommended by the American Heart Association (the average American eats more than 3,400 mg a day!).

Because plant-based diets tend to be naturally low in iodine (table salt is often "iodized salt"), you might want to drink a glass of water every day with a few drops of a liquid iodine supplement added in per the instructions on the bottle to be sure that you are getting adequate iodine in your diet, after checking with your health professional.

Remember the wildly successful "stop smoking campaign" from a few decades ago that saved countless lives through better awareness of the dangers of smoking? Perhaps our next national campaign should be a "stop salting campaign," which, if successful, would likewise save hundreds of thousands of lives every year from stroke and cardiovascular deaths that are attributable to dietary salt.

Does eating healthily build a strong immune system?

Based on my experience, I believe it does. Several of my grandchildren lived at my house for a good part of a summer. At one point, I watched as each of them came down with a stubborn sore throat, like a set of dominoes being toppled over one by one. Their sore throats later developed into colds. As my wife and I watched this, we expected that we would catch the virus ourselves. However, it didn't happen. I don't believe it was because we weren't exposed. Kids touch almost everything that others do in a house. We ate in the same kitchen, breathed the same air, played together, and shared the same environment. Rather, I believe it was because of our diet.

My wife swears that since she has been eating healthier by adhering to a plant-based diet and avoiding junk food, she has not had a cold. She said that previously, she was almost always sick with something, especially during cold season. The same thing happened to me.

Although this is anecdotal evidence, if it works for me, then I don't care if it fails to prove anything scientifically. Because of my own experience, I am convinced that eating healthily has made my immune systems significantly stronger. To me, it just makes sense that if I nourish my cells optimally, they will perform their best for me.

But you don't need to rely on my anecdotal experience. As Dr. Michael Greger has reported in his video, "Using the Produce Aisle to Boost Immune Function" on nutritionfacts.org, eating plant-based foods does indeed boost your immune system.

WEEK 18

"Isn't it fun to drive by fast food restaurants now without being tempted to make a stop?"

"This is to die for"

I sometimes wonder how the phrase, "This is to die for" originated. Would people really trade their lives for a morsel of cake or a piece of pie? I often hear chefs on their shows describing one of their desserts in this way only to find out that it is full of butter, cream, sugar, eggs, and white flour. Because of this, I wonder if they know they are speaking the truth much more profoundly than they realize.

Americans eat food all that time that "is to die for." The standard American diet (SAD) is full of fatty meat, dairy, eggs, salt, sugar, fast food, junk food, and highly processed packaged goods—things that taste good, but which are addictive, overstimulate our brains, lead to disease, and shorten our lifespans.

Perhaps a chef should instead prepare a scrumptious nutritarian entrée, dessert, or side dish and then exclaim, "This is to live for!" Healthy foods are full of life-giving micronutrients that deeply nourish the cells of your body and fight off disease. They help sustain life, thus validating this rephrased exclamation. Those who eat a whole-food, plant-based diet live longer and on average enjoy better health throughout their lives than those who eat the standard American diet.

When you fully understand the power of plants to bring you outstanding health and extend your life, you too will exclaim, whenever you eat healthy food, "This is to live for!"

Being penny wise and pound foolish

Some people shun buying "expensive" natural foods at the grocery store like raw, unsalted nuts or fresh or frozen berries, saying that such foods are just too expensive. These people then stroll down the grocery store aisles and load up their carts with meat, cheese, cookies, crackers, prepared breakfast cereals, candy, and ice cream, much of which is even more expensive per serving than whole, plant-based foods.

Take raw, unsalted cashews, for example, which is one of the most expensive whole, plant-based foods you can buy. They may seem expensive, even when you buy them in bulk at a farmer's market or at a big box store. You are not accustomed to paying that much for any one food item. But when you figure out that you are only using five or six nuts per day (as part of your daily mix of nuts), it turns out that your container of nuts lasts longer than the two or three cartons of ice cream you recently brought home.

The same goes for fresh fruit or frozen berries. You may think that a bag of apples or a carton of strawberries from the wholesale club is expensive, but when you eat just one apple and a few strawberries a day, they last several days. If you stop buying meat, dairy, eggs, cereal, cookies, crackers, chips, candy, soda, and other unhealthy foods, you would have plenty of money left over to buy healthy foods.

When you compare the price per pound for meat versus the price per pound for fresh fruit, you will see that meat costs four or five times more per pound than many fruits. Since most Americans eat a substantial serving of meat at both lunch and dinner, a large bag of pre-washed salad greens is cheap by comparison. Fresh, cut-up vegetables ("finger foods") also last for several meals. Dried beans and grains are very economical when bought in bulk, and you only need a small amount (before cooking) per serving size.

If you are stingy with buying real food, your health will suffer. You will have a weaker immune system. You will go to the doctor's office more often, and you will fill more prescriptions. Your copay alone for a couple of these visits might cost the same as buying fresh fruit for several weeks. And if you eventually develop a chronic disease because of your nutritional neglect, such as type 2 diabetes, kidney disease, or cardiovascular disease, your treatment and prescription costs will really tax your pocketbook. These are costs you might have to pay out monthly for the rest of your life.

So stop being penny wise and pound foolish. Buy healthy food—it is one of the best bargains (and investments) around.

Do we practice "healthcare" or "sickcare" in the U.S.?

According to Dr. Joel Fuhrman, we practice "sickcare"—not "healthcare"—in the U.S. (see *The End of Dieting*, p. 90), meaning almost all of our medical healthcare dollars go to treating the symptoms of disease instead of treating the causes of disease (prevention). He points out that we are already spending 20 percent of our gross domestic product (as of the publication date of his book, 2014) on healthcare, a figure that continues to rise, putting a strain on our economy that soon will become unsustainable.

We have relegated the responsibility for our health to people in white coats. We put our trust in doctors and hospitals to save us from our own personal health disasters brought on by years of neglect and nutritional self-abuse. We believe that if we just pay out enough money, these professionals will keep us healthy with their specialized knowledge, medicines, procedures, and high-tech medical equipment. And they are happy to try, taking a big bite out of our billfolds along the way. At the same time, we feel happy because we don't have to give our health a second thought and can go back to eating anything we want.

While this might seem like a beneficial symbiotic relationship, there is more to understand than first meets the eye. Treating the symptoms instead of the causes of disease means that, when we contract a serious disease:

- We undergo expensive and painful invasive procedures to treat the symptoms of the disease, including procedures such as angioplasty, by-pass surgery, stints, radiation, chemotherapy, dialysis, transplants, and tumor-and-organ-removal surgeries.
- The treatment seldom cures or addresses the cause of the disease, so we may be sick for the rest of our lives or suffer multiple future recurrences. For example, procedures such as artery stints and by-pass surgeries don't address the cause of the heart disease—they only treat the symptoms. The disease is still present, so future heart attacks or strokes are likely. This means we will have to endure the ongoing pains of the illness and its treatment for the foreseeable future and live in constant fear and anxiety that we will have another heart attack, stroke, or recurrence of cancer.
- We will have to take one or more expensive medications for the rest of our lives, taking more money out of our wallets and inflicting powerful side-effects on our bodies that we must endure in addition to the pains of our illness.
- We pass through one-way doors—our lives will never go back to "the way it was."
- Our personal freedoms, enjoyments, and capabilities in life are constrained due to the physical, mental, and emotional limitations imposed on us by the disease.
- The lives of our loved ones are changed. They have to cope with the threat of losing someone close to them and with the threat of losing their source of income or other contributions you might be

making. They may also have to deal with the burdens of being a caretaker.

To replace "sickcare" with "healthcare," we must change *who* we believe is responsible for our health, how we educate patients when they come down with a disease, and the industries we support or sustain with our tax dollars as part of public policy. Maybe it's time to stop beating at the leaves and get at the root of the problem.

Can we exercise our way out of the obesity crisis?

The federal government just updated its guidelines for physical activity for Americans in an effort to fight the obesity epidemic that affects 38 percent of Americans and adds nearly $117 billion to health care costs. In a sad commentary on our times, the new guidelines added, for the first time, recommendations that preschoolers 3- to 5-years old engage in physical activity for about three hours a day. Many preschoolers who start out overweight as children become obese as adults, and physical activity habits developed during childhood typically carry over into adulthood.

Although exercise in all its varieties is highly beneficial to our health (the report said that it helps prevent eight types of cancer), we are not going to exercise our way out of the obesity crisis. As reported by Dr. Michael Greger, a recent survey showed that the number of Americans who reported that they are eating "whatever they want" is at an all-time high and that Americans are eating far too few (and too little variety) of fruits and vegetables. And while gym and fitness center memberships have almost doubled from 2000 to 2017, obesity rates have steadily increased over that same period.

If the boat we are in is sinking, it makes sense to plug up the largest hole first. If the government were really serious about tackling the obesity crisis in this country, it should focus on what Americans are eating, not on how much exercise they are getting.

Controlling weight is all about eating real food and avoiding unhealthy food. It is very difficult for most people to control their weight while eating the standard American diet—a diet filled with junk foods, fast foods, and highly processed foods. These foods are addictive and full of things like added sugars, refined carbs, and fats that are quickly converted into fat on the body.

So, while Americans need to get moving, they more urgently need to start eating healthy foods and stop eating unhealthy foods. Only then can we hope to see improvements in both our health and our waistlines.

Dress for success

One of the nicest benefits of eating a whole-food, plant based diet, such as the nutritarian diet, is the weight loss that will occur naturally as a side benefit. When you eat the right foods, and only the right foods, you will fill your stomach at every meal with fewer calories, your body will be deeply nourished, "toxic hunger" will depart, and you will have greater willpower to avoid addictive, calorie-concentrated "artificial" foods that are full of added sugar, fat, refined carbs, and oils. Then, one day, you will wake up to a whole new problem—one you won't mind having—the need to buy smaller clothes.

When you go out on this exciting activity, be sure to choose clothing that makes you feel good about your "new you." Discard or donate the baggy clothing you wore in your previous life. Wear clothing that fits.

That way, when you look at yourself in the mirror wearing your new clothes, you will be proud of yourself and what you have accomplished. You will be motivated to keep things just the way they are. Instead of giving in to junk-food binges, you will think, "I'd rather keep my waistline exactly where it is than eat this fake food that will only give me temporary pleasure, bump up my weight, and injure my health."

Ignoring the legal fine print

Have legal notices that show up in our modern society encouraged us to ignore the possible serious consequences of our actions? For example, every time I install new software on my computer, I must check a box that says, "You have read and agree to the terms and conditions of this software." When I click the link to read the actual agreement, a long document is displayed that is filled with unending legalese that would make anyone's head swim. If you are like me, I sometimes check the box without reading the agreement so I can move forward with the installation.

Similarly, when drug companies advertise their products on TV, they rehearse a list of disclaimers that is often longer than the rest of the ad. These disclaimers include many startling statements, such as, "This product may cause seizures, internal bleeding, cancer, rashes, liver failure, stroke, heart attack, loss of vision, impaired cognition ..." and a host of other horrible possible side-effects, sometimes including death! How can anyone hear all these terrible things and still want to buy their product? Apparently they do, and marketers know it.

One simple explanation is that people group disclaimers into a separate mental category that they can easily dismiss or ignore as something that is very unlikely to happen to them, happens only rarely, or is only given for legal protection of the seller. When we know we are only one purchase or click away from enjoying the product, we click away without giving those possibilities a second thought.

Similarly, when we hear news reports, read magazine articles, or otherwise receive information that fast food, junk food, and processed food is harmful to our health and causes cancer, stroke, heart disease, obesity, type 2 diabetes, high blood pressure, cognitive impairment, early death, and a whole host of other serious diseases and health problems (see Dr. Joel Fuhrman's book, *Fast Food Genocide*), do we just brush them off like legal disclaimers, thinking they are exaggerations that are unlikely to happen to us or are consequences that rarely occur? Do we think we are safe because we observe others dismissing these dangers without incurring any detectable negative consequences?

Thoughtless actions lead to thought-filled regrets. We must not let our culturally trained impulse to click by all the disclaimers override our own careful intellectual assessments.

How valuable is your health?

As humans, we take things for granted until they are taken away from us. We erroneously think that Newton's first law of motion—"Things that are in motion will stay in motion unless acted upon by an external force"—applies not only to objects in space, but to our lives. For example, if we are currently enjoying good health—despite what we eat—we think that we will continue to enjoy good health indefinitely (or at least until we are "old"). It is only after our health fails that we develop a profound appreciation for what we previously had and find ourselves wishing we could turn back the clock. It has been said that "If you want to know how valuable your health is, just ask someone who has recently lost it."

A few winters ago, I fell down some icy steps and broke my wrist. Aside from the pain of the injury and the expense of treating it, my entire arm was immobilized in a soft cast, which limited my actions to using only one hand and arm. Because of this, I developed a whole new appreciation for having two functioning arms and hands to perform basic daily tasks. I also learned to walk more cautiously on icy surfaces.

Although my loss was temporary, not all health losses are reversible. You can pass through "one-way doors" for which there is no return, where no amount of money, surgery, medications, physical therapy, or remorse will bring back the health you once enjoyed. All you can do is to live with your regrets, restrictions, and pain and warn others to avoid a similar fate, like Jacob Marley in "The Christmas Carol." Unfortunately, such advice typically falls on deaf ears or uninterested or distracted minds, leaving others to learn for themselves just how valuable their health is—by losing it.

Your body is the only tool you have by which you can interact with the external world and do the things in life you want to do. Moreover, it houses your brain, which allows you to think and solve problems. If you want to develop your unique talents, express your creativity, earn a living, raise a family, and enjoy the finer things in life, you will need a body. But you only get one body in this life. You cannot abuse it, throw it away, and then buy another one, like some worn-out old car.

So, how do you want to learn to value your health—through losing it, or by witnessing what its loss has done to others and learn from their experiences?

WEEK 19

"You are a sterling example of someone who eats healthily."

Does misery motivate change?

Whenever I leave the dentist's office, I feel a renewed resolve to take excellent care of my teeth. The experience of laying in the dentist's chair getting a root canal, filling, or a crown motivates me to change. The pain, the inconvenience, the time, and the financial cost all have a way of getting my brain's attention. For the next several days, I brush immediately after eating and floss my teeth religiously every night. Over time, though, the memory of my pain starts to fade and old habits sometimes begin to reappear unless I am careful to consciously intervene.

It has been said that addicts often have to "bottom out" before they become serious about overcoming their addictions. Only when they are miserable enough or suffer a traumatic event, such as having a friend or loved one die from an overdose, will they consider making the painful journey to overcome their addictions. Of course, there are some drug addicts who will never change, even in the face of death.

Are we like that when it comes to our food addictions? Do we dismiss the need to change our diet until the day our habits catch up with us and we find ourselves laying on a hospital gurney with our sternum cracked open having open-heart surgery or find ourselves in a hospital bed with an IV bag attached to us that is dripping toxic chemotherapy drugs into our bloodstream? Why do we wait until after our health has failed, after we are in acute pain, or after our lives are turned upside down before we will consider changing our ways? Are we one of those people who will never change—even in the face of extreme pain and misery—choosing instead to let our addictions ultimately take our lives, just as with some drug addicts?

While it may be human nature to satisfy our addictions until we crash and burn, we are not totally under the control of our instincts, as is the rest of the animal kingdom. We are different because we have self-awareness, and we have agency, which is the ability to consciously intervene and select a path of our own choosing that is different from that dictated by our instincts. Because of this, we don't have to wait until pain and misery destroy our happy reality to change. We can look into the future and see negative consequences *before* they happen, if we have the eyes to see. Then, we can use wisdom to choose a different path.

So, don't let pain and misery be your only teacher. Take advantage of your unique human qualities in the animal kingdom. Allow nutritional education to enlighten you so that you can see the oncoming train wreck before it happens and switch to a different, healthier track of your own choosing.

Make your home a "safe house" for healthy living

Everyone knows that people who have addictions should not live in an environment that constantly tests their resolve to stay "clean." Alcoholics should not keep alcohol stashed away in their closets. Drug addicts should not keep drugs hidden under their bed pillows. Gambling addicts should not have access to unblocked gambling websites on their computers. Instead, the living environment of addicts should be "substance-free zones"—places that are devoid of the temptations that could send them spiraling back down the black hole of addiction.

Similarly, because fast food, junk food, and processed food contain refined carbs, sugar, fat, and salt—things that are known to have strong addictive qualities (just try to give up junk food for a month and see how the addiction centers of your brain react)—if you are serious about converting over to healthy eating, you must make your home a "junk-food-free" zone.

To do this requires that you first clear out all the unhealthy foods from your pantry, refrigerator, and freezer. This means everything, including dairy products (ice cream, yogurt, milk, and cheese), meats, eggs, cooking oils, cookies, crackers, chips, candies, prepared breakfast cereals, cake mixes, muffin mixes, white flour bins, pancake mixes and syrup, juices, white and brown sugar, white rice, sports drinks, and soft drinks. Second, you must restock your home with healthy, plant-based alternatives, such as fresh and frozen fruits and vegetables, whole grains, beans (and other legumes), raw nuts, and seeds that can be eaten plain or used in recipes that only use these ingredients.

When doing this, you must be ruthless. Sugar addicts have a way of finding any food that was overlooked that would give them another dopamine high. Not only must you get rid of foods that have added sugar in them (in all of its forms), you must get rid of foods that have ingredients in them that quickly convert into sugar in the digestive tract, like white pasta, white bread, and other foods made with white flour, white rice, white potatoes, or other highly refined grains or carbohydrates. You must also carefully scrutinize your canned and packaged goods to see if they have any unhealthful ingredients.

Do your "house cleaning" as part of an overall, well-thought-out plan for transitioning to healthy eating—not as an impulsive, spur-of-the-moment, Storm-Trooper-style siege. This will better prepare you to endure the withdrawal phase of addiction. As part of that preparation, build up your collection of healthy recipes and your skill in preparing them so you can replace unhealthy food with healthy food.

Society has set aside bird refuges and sanctuaries as places where birds are safe from being shot or otherwise being harmed. Why not create your own "food sanctuary" where you can be safe from being brought down by destructive and harmful "fake foods" that otherwise would tempt you?

Living free of food addictions

Before I changed my diet to a whole-food, plant-based diet, I lived with what Joel Fuhrman calls "toxic hunger"—constant junk-food cravings, a false sense of hunger soon after eating, and inadequate nutrition (meaning insufficient antioxidants and phytonutrients). When late evening came, I needed my daily fix of chips, ice cream, buttered popcorn, cake, or chocolate chip cookies just to wind down for the day. I loved all kinds of unhealthy foods—junk foods, processed foods, fast foods—anything that tasted good. During workdays, I would often daydream about stopping at the grocery store on the way home to pick up some "treats."

But since I have adopted a nutritarian diet—one consisting of whole grains, fruits, vegetables, legumes, cooked mushrooms, nuts, spices, and seeds—and nothing else—my body has since been healed of nutritional deficiencies, my cravings have subsided, my blood-sugar levels have stabilized, my energy level has increased, my waistline has decreased, my true hunger signals have reappeared, and my overall health has greatly improved. No longer am I haunted every night by thoughts of eating junk food nor do I feel compelled to make a "junk-food run" to the local convenience store.

Being free of food addictions is liberating. My mental and emotional energies are totally available to pursue other, more worthy, goals. My reliance on food as an emotional crutch has subsided. My pocketbook has more money in it from the junk-food purchases I never made. My freedom to walk down the grocery store aisles without being captured by the siren songs of unhealthy food is secure. My body is lighter, more athletic looking, and better able to accomplish physical tasks. Finally, I feel at peace knowing that I am treating my body with the respect it deserves, feeding it only foods that nourish it and doing it no harm. These are all rewards for healthy eating—in addition to better health!

Food addictions are no myth. Breaking free of them is a challenge of a lifetime, but once you have conquered them, you will likely never want to give up your freedom again for a few temporary pleasures and a long-term addiction to unhealthy and harmful food.

How healthy eating becomes self-motivating

If you consistently eat healthy foods—and only healthy foods—eventually, healthy eating will become self-motivating. You will want to continue eating this way because:

- You will experience how great you feel physically, mentally, and emotionally,
- Your taste buds will change—you will find whole, plant-based foods and recipes delicious and satisfying,
- You will notice that you don't get sick as often,
- Your intense cravings for junk food will subside,
- Your energy level will become more even,
- You will shed excess weight, and
- You will notice that many of your existing health issues actually go away!

In short, no one will have to sell you on why you should eat healthily. As far as you are concerned, you have proven the benefits to yourself. To you, they are established facts. All of the criticisms over "flaws" in nutritional research, all of the debate over what is healthy and what isn't, all of the uncertainty created by the promoters and purveyors of unhealthy food will simply no longer be of any concern. For you, the matter will be a closed book.

It's almost as if you were a castaway on a tropical island who had discovered a pool of fresh water surrounded by groves of mango, banana, and date trees while those back on the beach are hungrily debating over whether fresh water and fruit trees could exist on the island. While you are drinking cool, clear water and eating fresh, luscious fruit, they are stuck arguing whether such a scenario exists, while at the same time, refusing to make the effort to hike to the pool to see for themselves.

What is amazing is that these benefits can be replicated by anyone who is willing to perform the experiment. It's not just a lucky few who are granted improved health and other benefits—it is almost *anyone* who is willing to make the change. This is a proposition that passes the test of reality, a true cause-and-effect relationship. Those who pay the price of healthy eating get the benefits. Those who don't, don't. It's as simple as that. If you are willing to change your diet, the debate ends there. For those who aren't, debate on!

"Fan food—not fast food"

When fast-food marketers sense that their product's name is falling out of favor because people are starting to realize how unhealthy their products are, they pull a fast one—they change the name of their product or how it is called to a more socially acceptable one. Amazingly, it works, and they don't even have to change their product. I saw this happen again last week when a TV commercial for a major fast food chain that sells burgers, fries, soda, and ice cream touted that they now sell "fan food—not fast food."

But how can "fan food" not be "fast food" if it is still the same product? If the food is just as unhealthy as it ever was, then it still is "fast food." Just because marketers dub their product with a healthier-sounding name doesn't mean it is healthier. If you eat it, it will still do to your body exactly what it did before.

So, how can people fall for such obvious tactics? It's not because they are stupid. Rather, I believe it is because people want to continue eating fast food and *feel good* about doing it. In other words, they willingly allow themselves to be seduced by marketing messages that help dispel the cognitive dissonance they are feeling. They experience these uncomfortable feelings when they know that what they are currently eating—fast food—is not what they should be eating to have long-term health.

Moreover, when junk-food marketers can't change the facts about their products, they try to change how people *feel* about their products (in marketing, it's all about the *feeling*, not the *reality*). Junk-food marketers have become masters at manipulating feelings. They can make us feel good about uncomfortable truths by failing to mention them or glossing over them with catchy tag lines, attractive names, appealing jingles, celebrity endorsements, visually stimulating videos, snippets of people enjoying their products as part of the good life, and above all, never showing any negative consequences of consuming their products.

Advertisements for cigarettes, for example, tried to associate their product with movie stars, with "high society," with "being a real man or woman," with doctors' endorsements, and even with good health (I had to see those ads to believe it). But their product was still as deadly as ever. Putting a pretty label on a cyanide bottle or a carton of cigarettes does not make their contents any less deadly. It only makes those who use them feel better while using them. The consequences are the same.

So, don't let junk-food purveyors with their clever tactics damage your health. You must not only be "buyer beware," but "eater beware."

Are plant-based diets the nutritional equivalent of quitting smoking?

According to an editorial published in the American Medical Association Journal of Ethics by Dr. Neal Barnard, associate professor of medicine at the George Washington University School of Medicine and Health Sciences and the founder of the Physicians Committee for Responsible Medicine, the answer to this question is "yes." Indeed, many nutrition researchers and studies have concluded that the number one cause of death today is diet and lifestyle. We are killing ourselves by what we are putting on our forks, just as we were killing ourselves by what we held between our lips in the heyday of cigarette smoking.

Unfortunately, while almost everyone in today's society views cigarette smoking as extremely dangerous to one's health, few people see eating the standard American diet (SAD) in the same light. Rather, most people choose what they eat based on how good food tastes or how good it makes them feel, not on how well it nourishes their body. But if you carefully read Dr. Barnard's statement, it is not the addition of an apple-a-day that is going to do the trick. It is eating a *plant*-based diet. This is a diet that is plant-based and that avoids all animal products and other unhealthy foods.

Just as smokers did not want to hear in their day that smoking might be bad for their health, people today don't want to hear that eating meat, eggs, and dairy products are bad for them:

- It doesn't matter that the World Health Organization has classified processed meats as Group 1 carcinogens and red meat as Group 2 carcinogens (the worst categories).
- It doesn't matter that the protein in meat (but not plant protein) has been shown to increase levels in humans of the cancer-promoting growth hormone IGF-1 and to promote the formation of TMAO in the liver—a "molecule from hell" that drives cholesterol into your artery walls.
- It doesn't matter if meat promotes the "bad bacteria" instead of the "good bacteria" in your gut that plays such an important role in your health.
- It doesn't matter if tests of meat have been found to sometimes contain banned drugs, carcinogenic chemicals, antibiotics, and other harmful substances.
- It doesn't matter if meat is loaded with cholesterol and saturated fat that cause artery and heart disease, high blood pressure, and other serious diseases.
- It doesn't matter if animal products are responsible for many of the *48 million* people who get sick from foodborne illnesses every year in the U.S., resulting in 128,000 hospitalizations and 3,000 deaths.
- It doesn't matter if you can get all the protein your body needs simply by eating a variety of plant-based fruits, vegetables, legumes, whole grains, nuts, and seeds.
- It doesn't matter that nutrition researchers have called milk products "liquid meat" and stated that they are just as bad (or even worse) for your health as eating meat.

It doesn't matter if the many phytonutrients that are being discovered every year that are found to be essential to fighting cell oxidation, killing cancerous cells, arresting and slowing cell aging and cellular death, and maintaining cellular health and function are found only in plants.

Someday society will view the eating of meat, eggs, and dairy products as dangerous to one's health as smoking cigarettes. They will also view the eating of a plant-based diet as just as important. But why wait until then to start protecting your health? Go "smoke free" today by switching to a plant-based diet.

You are in truth what you eat

I recently saw a pizza commercial on TV showing a close-up of the faces of a young couple drooling over a large pizza in an oven. After a brief conversation, the young lady suddenly jumps back, revealing that she is wearing pajamas with images of round pepperoni slices all over them from top to bottom. She then exclaims, "You are what you eat!" and the commercial abruptly ends.

I thought to myself, "This commercial speaks the truth more than it realizes." This lady's body is in part made up of greasy pepperoni (a Group 1 carcinogen full of saturated fat); fatty, addictive, cholesterol-laden cheese; pizza sauce containing generous portions of sugar, salt, and cooking oil; and pizza dough containing refined white flour, more salt, and dough enhancers and additives.

Although we have all heard the phrase "you are what you eat," it seems that many of us don't seem to grasp what that really means—or at least don't seem to care about its implications. To me, it means that the only material my body—my skin, bones, organs, brain cells, nerves, blood vessels, and blood—has for cell reproduction, growth, repair, operation, and disease prevention, is what I eat. It all comes from those few morsels of food I consume every day.

Of course, your body doesn't magically sustain itself on thin air as some people apparently seem to think. It must be nourished by something, and that something is the total collection of molecules in the food you eat. These molecules not only maintain existing cells, they provide the raw material your body needs to create new cells when your old cells die. Most of the cells in your body are replaced every few months or years, which means you are literally re-creating your body every so often from the inside out. The only question is, out of what?

Since it is difficult to view the actual molecules you eat with the naked eye, suppose you were to lay out on a table all the ingredients that make up the food you are currently eating—the refined white flours, the chemical powders, the food coloring, the liquid sweeteners, the refined oils, the piles of salt and added sugars, and the AGF-1-hormone-inducing, toxin-and pesticide-contaminated animal products you eat (as reported in a recent issue of a leading consumer magazine). Do you really believe that these bland powders; calorie-laden, nutrient-deficient liquids; and disease-promoting animal products will provide your body with what it needs to produce health and longevity and fight off disease? Do you really believe that these ingredients were invented by modern technology to *enhance nutrition*, or can you consider the possibility that they were created to *enhance the pocketbooks* of those who manufacture and sell these products and extend shelf life?

If our bodies could speak, I wonder what they would say:

- "Do you really expect me to maintain this most complex marvel of all biological life with the 'fake food' you are feeding me?"
- "Hey, man [or woman]. It's junk in, junk out. It's your choice—but I can't produce quality results when you feed me junky food."
- "Why aren't you feeding me all the phytonutrients, fiber, resistant starches, and antioxidants that my cells and my gut are crying out for that are found only in whole, unrefined, plant-based foods—foods I was designed to eat?"
- "How can I keep you cancer free, diabetes free, heart-attack free, stroke free, arthritis free, and clogged-artery free when you are feeding me *junk* as my building material?"

If we are what we eat, then many people are not what they seem to be. Instead, they are carrying around compromised bodies that are prone to cancer, heart disease, kidney disease, type 2 diabetes, stroke, and other health issues—problems that will almost certainly exact a heavy toll at some point in their future lives.

As for myself, I want my body to like me for what I eat, and I want to like how my body treats me in return. That's why I choose to eat only nutrient-dense, whole, plant-based foods.

So, for the sake of your body, don't fall into the trap of selecting food based solely on its pleasure value. Instead, select food based on its micronutrient value. Your body will love you for it, and you, in turn, will love your body.

WEEK 20

"The summit approaches! Aren't you proud of yourself? You should be!"

Going nuts over nuts

I can't imagine my whole-food, plant-based diet without raw, unsalted nuts and seeds. I eat ground up flax, sesame, and chia seeds as part of my breakfast and a variety of raw, unsalted nuts (almonds, walnuts, pecans, cashews, pistachios, and a Brazil nut) and seeds (pumpkin, hemp, and sunflower) with my lunch and dinner. They are a real treat to eat, and I savor every bite. I don't really feel satisfied at lunch and dinner until after I have eaten a handful of nuts and seeds. This is probably because nuts and seeds have healthy fats in them that help me feel satiated and that slow the digestion of my meal, keeping my energy levels stable in-between meals.

But that's not all that nuts and seeds have to offer. They are chock-full of protein, antioxidants, minerals, fiber, complex carbohydrates, and beneficial micronutrients, such as plant sterols, which help reduce cholesterol and reduce the risk of cancer. Some (including flaxseeds, hemp seeds, chia seeds, and walnuts) are rich in omega-3 fatty acids, which promote heart and brain health.

As reported by Dr. Michael Greger (see his book, *How Not to Die*) and Dr. Joel Fuhrman (see his book, *The End of Dieting*), according to the available research, eating nuts and seeds can:

- Extend your life by about two years,
- Lower your cholesterol levels, especially the "bad" LDL cholesterol, with no ill side effects,
- Protect you against cancer, including breast and prostate cancer, especially when you eat flax, chia, and sesame seeds, which are rich in lignans (note that flaxseeds must be ground up to be digested),
- Cut your risk of stroke, cancer, and heart disease in half by eating walnuts and other nuts and seeds,
- Increase the absorption of the beneficial phytochemicals and antioxidants in dark, leafy greens and vegetables up to ten-fold when eaten at the same time,
- Help stabilize blood glucose levels, and
- Lead to fewer deaths from cancer, heart disease, and respiratory disease.

Shockingly, according to the Global Burden of Disease Study, not eating enough nuts and seeds was listed as the third-leading dietary risk factor for death and disability *in the world*.

So, what's not to like? The benefits listed above of extending your life by two years and cutting your risk in half for getting common diseases such as cancer, stroke, and heart disease—all without any side effects—should make it worth your trouble of eating a few nuts and seeds every day, even if you don't change your diet in any other way. People would pay big bucks for a pill that did that, and even if it existed, it would likely be accompanied by a list of serious possible side effects that was a mile long.

Worried that eating nuts and seeds will increase your weight? Numerous studies have shown that eating nuts and seeds does not cause weight gain when a handful or two are added to your diet. Just eat them with your meals so you will absorb more of the beneficial micronutrients in your salads and vegetables and slow the digestion of your food. Avoid indiscriminately eating them like popcorn for snacks, which will lead to weight gain, and avoid eating nuts that are roasted in oils or fats.

Garbage collection day for your cells

Whenever you consume things like sugar, white bread, white pasta, white potatoes, candy, soda, French fries, or other junk food that quickly dumps a huge load of sugar into your bloodstream, your pancreas shifts into overdrive and releases a corresponding amount of insulin. When the cells of your body finally metabolize this huge sugar load, they create toxic metabolites. If you haven't eaten a corresponding influx of micronutrients to counteract and "clean up the garbage," these metabolites can wreak havoc to the cells in your body (see p. 53 in Dr. Joel Fuhrman's book, *The End of Dieting*).

In other words, consuming pure calories without also consuming the antioxidants and phytochemicals found in plants allows these harmful metabolites in your cells to do their damage unchecked. It's like garbage pickup day for your cells never comes and the garbage piles up day after day. A buildup of these toxic metabolites can eventually help promote disease. For example, studies have shown that high-glycemic, low-nutrient foods (such as sugar and highly refined carbohydrates, such as flour and white rice) are linked to cancer. Plants are the only source for getting these valuable phytochemicals.

This is just one more reason that eating junk food is bad for your health. You're much better off getting your calories from whole, plant-based foods where you intake not only calories, but the antioxidants and phytonutrients to metabolize these calories safely.

So, the next time you eat that hamburger and fries and gulp down that soda, visualize the toxic metabolites that are building up in your cells and the overall cellular stress you are putting your body through. It's garbage in, garbage stays, and garbage rots (does damage).

How much uncollected garbage do you have in your cells?

Is what you see what you get?

When you look at others, do you judge how healthy they are by their appearance? Is what you see a good indicator of their overall health? For example, if they look healthy and you don't see any visible signs of illness, do you conclude that they are in good health?

If this is true, then nearly everyone around you is healthy because most people *look* healthy. Health must be the norm, even though people are running around indulging in eating whatever they want, stuffing their faces with hamburgers, pizza, ice cream, processed meats, cheese, eggs, candy, cookies, cakes, soda, chips, and donuts. Despite what they eat, they still appear to be healthy.

This, however, cannot be the true. Why? Consider the following:

- One-third of all Americans are classified as obese (according to The Journal of the American Medical Association—JAMA), and that percentage is expected to soar over the next several years.
- About 1 in 7 Americans have type 2 diabetes, and that number is expected to top 1 in 3 in just a couple of decades.
- One-fourth or more Americans have fatty liver disease, with many people unaware that they even have the disease.
- If you believe the top 15 leading causes of death in the U.S., the majority of Americans are silently but steadily progressing toward heart disease, kidney disease, cancer, stroke, and a host of other serious health problems.

A person's skin is only a few cells deep and accounts for only 15 percent of a person's body weight. The human body contains dozens of other organs, bones, tissues, and cells that must all work perfectly and harmoniously for good health. Just because you can't see what's going on "behind the scenes" does not mean that nothing is happening. What you see is not what you get.

And that's a big part of the problem. When we see others eating junk food at will with no immediate, visible consequences to their health, we don't see the need to change what we are eating. We believe our own eyes, and we find comfort in following the crowd. We don't want to believe the impressive data that shows that 80 to 90 percent of most of our leading causes of death are preventable through diet. So, we "free ourselves of the facts" and then conclude that now is the time to enjoy the good life—along with everyone else—by eating food that is fun, highly rewarding, and addictive. We can feel guiltless about eating ourselves to death.

But what if we lived in a world in which the consequences of eating junk were immediately visible on your body. What if your skin suddenly broke out with boils after eating a greasy hamburger or if you started coughing up blood after eating a couple of slices of pizza? What if you starting having severe chest pains and gasping for breath after you ate a big steak with a "loaded" baked potato. What if your body had some way of visibly signaling to you that the food you are eating is harmful? Would you then take your diet more seriously? Your body is a silent victim, so use your knowledge of nutrition to choose what you eat, not your taste buds or your food addictions.

The lowdown on antioxidant-laden legumes

Legumes (beans, peas, chickpeas, and lentils) are one of the healthiest, most beneficial foods around. They are chock-full of protein, fiber, antioxidants, minerals, vitamins, slowly-digestible starch, and many other beneficial nutrients. One of their many stellar qualities is that they contain an *abundance* of antioxidants.

Antioxidants neutralize free radicals—molecules produced when your body breaks down food or is exposed to tobacco smoke or radiation. Free radicals are unstable molecules that lack an electron in their outer shell, which causes them to seek to bind with another electron. They can damage DNA and other cellular structures and can even form chain reactions in which the molecules they damage also turn into free radicals.

Antioxidant molecules can give up a free electron, thus effectively neutralizing a free radical. Because free radicals are constantly being formed during metabolism, without antioxidants, they would quickly wreak havoc to the cells of our body. Getting your antioxidants in whole food rather than in isolated supplements, though, is important. The sum of the parts (the benefits) is always greater in whole foods than when singled out, extracted, and made into a supplement.

A study was conducted to compare the total antioxidant content of 10 different legumes (as reported in the video, "Benefits of Lentils and Chickpeas," on Dr. Michael Greger's website, nutritionfacts.org). Lentils came out on the very top as having the most antioxidants. Then, in descending order, came chickpeas, small red beans, black beans, pinto beans, red kidney beans, mung beans, black eye peas, navy beans, and last, lima beans.

Legumes provide other benefits besides antioxidants. They keep your stomach from emptying as quickly into your intestine, keeping you full longer and thus helping with appetite control. They feed the "good" bacteria in your gut, which are so crucial to your immune system and overall good health. They contain a lot of fiber, which has a number of health benefits. They are an excellent source of plant-based protein. They contain zinc, iron, magnesium, and folate. They reduce your chances of getting coronary heart disease, cancer, fatty liver disease, colon cancer, and Type 2 diabetes. They help to reduce your blood pressure. In short, from a health perspective, when you consider legumes, what's not to like?

Note: Beans *must* be completely cooked before they are eaten. Never eat beans raw.

Weight-loss drug brags about losing one negative side effect

On the national news recently, they proudly reported that a weight-loss drug no longer had the side effect of possibly causing heart disease. Imagine that! One side effect that could possibly kill you has been removed! They did not mention how many other side effects were still associated with the drug. The report mentioned that over 1in every 3 Americans are now overweight or obese.

According to Stephanie Winn of the American Cancer Society, 20 percent of all cancers are tied to being overweight.

California is taking legislative action to help prevent childhood obesity. A bill that limits restaurants to serving children water or unflavored milk with their meals was placed on the Governor's desk during the summer of 2018. Parents could still order alternative beverages, though, for their children. The CDC has linked frequent soda consumption with obesity, Type 2 diabetes, heart disease, kidney disease, nonalcoholic liver disease, tooth decay and cavities.

Is there a weight-loss method that has no adverse side effects other than making you healthier, in addition to losing weight? Yes! It's called eating a whole-food, plant based diet and avoiding animal products, refined carbs and oils, foods with added sugar, candies, and other junk foods. When I made the switch, I lost 45 pounds and have kept those pounds off since.

Meatless burgers

On the national news, I saw a story on meatless burgers, spotlighting a company that makes plant-based burgers intended to mimic the taste, texture, and flavor of real meat. Some restaurants even offer the burger on their menus, and a number of grocery stores are carrying the product in the refrigerated meat section. However, one nutritionist they interviewed in the news story was concerned that, even though the product is plant-based, it is made from *highly processed* plant-based ingredients.

My curiosity led me to their website to take a closer look at the ingredients listing and Nutrition Facts table. The first four ingredients were water, pea protein isolate, expeller-pressed canola oil, and refined coconut oil. The remaining ingredients were cellulose from bamboo, methylcellulose, potato starch, natural flavor, maltodextrin, yeast extract, salt, sunflower oil, vegetable glycerin, dried yeast, gum arabic, citrus extract (to protect quality), ascorbic acid (to maintain color), beet juice extract (for color), acetic acid, succinic acid, modified food starch, annatto (for color). So you be the judge—is this product made from whole plant foods or *highly processed* plant–based ingredients?

My other concern is they added a ton of fat back into the burgers with three kinds of processed vegetable oils. Vegetable oils have no nutrition to speak of and are 100 percent fat (9 calories per gram versus 4 calories for carbohydrates and proteins). More than 60 percent of the calories of their burgers comes from fat (170 out of 270), including 5 grams of saturated fat. Their burgers also have significant added salt (sodium) at 380 mg per serving and only 3 grams of fiber. So, while I believe that eating their burgers is much healthier than eating real hamburger meat, which is an animal product, they are still made from highly refined ingredients and are full of vegetable oil (a fat).

Instead of buying commercial meatless burgers, why not make your own hamburger-meat-substitute patties out of whole, plant-based ingredients? You can find many recipes for meatless burgers on websites such as www.ForksOverKnives.com or by searching for "meatless burger recipes" in your browser. While these substitutes are definitely different from regular hamburger meat patties, I have found that once you put them in a whole-wheat bun, add lettuce, onion, pickles, and other healthy condiments, they make a decent "burger" and are pretty palatable.

I applaud this company for making a meatless burger, but I think their goal of replicating the taste, texture, and flavor of real meat forced them into a corner of producing a highly refined product that still has lots of fat—just not animal fat. Instead, our goal ought to be to change our taste preferences toward eating whole-food, plant-based products.

Which organs of your body do you want to keep?

My dentist has a sign on the wall in front of each dental chair that says, "You don't have to brush all your teeth—only the ones you want to keep." That got me thinking. Perhaps we should hang a sign in corporate cafeterias, school lunch rooms, medical offices, and our homes that says, "You don't have to nourish all the organs of your body—only the ones you want to keep." Maybe that would get people to give a second thought to what they are putting into their mouths (other than their toothbrushes).

Every time you pick up your fork, you have the opportunity either to feed the organs of your body nutrient-dense food or feed them nutrient-deficient food. While your organs can forgive occasional nutritional mischief, they do have their limits. For example, nonalcoholic fatty liver disease is estimated to affect up to 25 percent of people in the U.S. It has been linked with being overweight or obese, having diabetes (or being insulin resistant), having high blood sugar, and having high levels of fat in your blood (especially triglycerides). These are all things that are associated with eating the standard American diet (SAD) year after year.

Moreover, nutrient-deficient foods release free radicals when they are metabolized that do cellular damage if they are not neutralized by the antioxidants and phytonutrients that are found in abundance in plant-based foods.

So, the next time you reach for that fast food meal or junk food snack, ask yourself, "Which organs of my body am *I* willing to give up?"

WEEK 21

"Aren't you glad you made the journey?"

Is trial-and-error all you need to guide your life?

Some of us believe our own wisdom, intuition, and experience are all we need to get by in life. While this belief is particularly strong in teenagers, adults can manifest it as well. Such individuals turn a deaf ear to the accumulated wisdom and experience of others who have identified valuable cause-and-effect relationships, such as what leads to pain, suffering, and loss of freedom and what leads to health, vitality, and lasting joy. Like rebellious teenagers who take up smoking, these people just want to be left alone so they can drive down life's road without anyone telling them "how to live their life" or warning them about upcoming hazards and consequences.

Imagine how far our civilization would advance if every new generation of engineers, doctors, tradespeople, and business entrepreneurs had to learn everything by trial-and-error, with nothing being passed on from generation to generation. What if parents failed to pass on their accumulated wisdom to their children and instead required their offspring to learn everything solely by trial-and-error? What if a novice mountain climber decided to climb Mt Everest without an experienced guide or mountaineering team?

As with most things in life, we cannot afford to take an "eat and see" approach with our diet. This is because we are biologically wired to eat foods based on how they look, smell, or taste. In today's modern food jungle, we naturally choose to eat foods that are full of fat, sugar, and salt. These artificially produced foods overstimulate the pleasure centers of the brain, lead to addiction, and promote obesity and disease. Because of this, we cannot just "eat what we want" for a lifetime and then "wait and see" what happens. If we do, we risk losing our health, our freedom, and even our lives.

Fortunately, we don't have to adopt this attitude. We can capitalize on the accumulated wisdom of others—decades of research that tells us that eating a whole-food, plant-based diet and avoiding junk foods, fast foods, and highly processed foods will bring us the greatest health and longevity and the most freedom from disease.

So, do you want to learn the hard way on your own, or do you want to access the accumulated wisdom of others to live the healthiest, most energetic, most productive life you can?

Get moving

I once attended a healthy lifestyle class at a local whole-grain food co-op. The instructor made the point that while you are working in the kitchen, you can use it as an opportunity to move and stretch your muscles while you cook, do dishes, or sweep the floor. Because of that insight, I now see working in the kitchen in an entirely different light. I am the one who ends up getting the most benefit. All that bending over, squatting, walking, stretching, and using my arms and legs helps keep me physically flexible and active. The same applies for other housework, such as vacuuming, mopping, doing laundry, and cleaning windows. Instead of viewing it as a burden, look at it as an opportunity to get some exercise and stretch your muscles.

I never complain about going up and down the three flights of stairs in my house because it feels so good to use my legs throughout the day. When I am out shopping, I try to park at the far end of the parking lot (where I can pull forward when I leave) to force me to walk some extra steps.

There are many ways to get moving—sports, dance, yoga, walking. I love to hike in the mountains, and I go every chance I get. You may have access to and love other sports and activities.

After consulting with your doctor or other medical professional, if you are healthy enough, consider starting a physical exercise routine at home or the gym or some other physical activity. The benefits of exercise on health are well known. Take the hard road physically. Do things that require physical exertion. Challenge yourself. Push through the inertia. Get moving!

Is "clean" food healthy food?

It seems like the latest marketing buzzword for selling fast food is pointing out that it is "clean" from a few unhealthy ingredients, such as preservatives or additives. Because "clean" is naturally associated with "wholesome" and "good," marketers accomplish their purpose of getting us to feel good about eating what they are selling, which leads to increased sales.

But can a food be labelled as healthy because of what it does *not* contain? I can sell you pure white sugar as "clean" food because it does not contain any harmful additives, but does that make refined sugar a healthy food? Remember to evaluate foods based on two criteria, not one, and in this order:

- Is this a nutrient-dense food (a whole, plant-based food)?

- Is this food free of added ingredients or toxins that are harmful or unhealthy?

In other words, does this food truly nourish my body without doing it any harm? If the food is not nutritious to begin with, then you should dismiss eating it, regardless of whether it carries with it any additional unhealthy "baggage" that makes it "unclean."

Beware of marketers who are master magicians in getting unhealthy food to appear as healthy food. Choose to eat only healthy food, not unhealthy food dressed up as "clean" food.

Are you too busy to take care of your body?

Where does taking care of your body fall in your list of daily priorities? Are you too busy to floss your teeth every day or even brush your teeth after every meal? Do you exercise daily? Do you stay on top of your athlete's foot infection? Do you go in for an annual physical? Do you eat junk food and fast food regularly?

In other words, do you shortchange taking care of your body to gain a few more measly minutes every day to do things you find more rewarding, such as watching television, socializing on social media, spending time with friends, or pursuing hobbies or entertainment? Do you really think you can cheat on caring for your body without any real consequences?

But consequences always follow. Failing to floss and brush your teeth can lead to serious gum disease and dental decay, causing eventual loss of teeth, bone, and the ability to chew. Lack of exercise contributes to obesity, heart disease, and other chronic diseases. Ignoring athlete's foot leads to thick and yellow toenails that are permanently infected by toenail fungus, possibly requiring toenail removal. Procrastination of annual physicals can lead to failing to detect the early signs of cancer or heart disease. Regularly eating fast food, junk food, and processed food increases your odds of living a shorter life and suffering many serious diseases and health problems.

We always seem to be in a hurry to rush through the "harder" things in life to get to the "fun things" we really enjoy. To counter this, slow down and learn to *enjoy* taking care of your body instead of seeing bodily care as an annoyance to be avoided, minimized, or shortchanged. Only when you respect your body and discipline yourself to care for it properly will you enjoy a greater sense of pride and have a body that is healthier, fitter, and more vibrant. By taking care of the truly important things in life, they, in turn, will help take care of you.

How many ways are there to justify buying and eating junk food?

In today's modern food culture, you are constantly bombarded with pleas to eat tempting junk food—from your kids when you drive by a fast food restaurant, from an ad on television for a candy bar, or from strolling down one of the many junk food aisles of your local grocery store. Impulses might even originate from your own thoughts when you remember the pleasures of your most recent junk-food encounter. All of these things tempt you to eat what you know is unhealthy.

At these times, your incredible human brain can be your own worst enemy. For example, if you really want to eat an ice cream sundae, it can invent a million reasons why you are justified in doing so:

- "I've had a hard day, so I deserve a treat as a reward."
- "It's Friday night—time to celebrate."
- "My emotions are in shambles. I need to self-soothe."
- "A little treat isn't a big deal."
- "No one's watching."
- "I promise myself I'll only eat one or two."
- "Look at others. They're loading up on junk food."
- "My body is strong. I can handle it."
- "I exercised this morning. I can afford the calories."
- "I have to buy this for a party or celebration."
- "It's organic, so it must be healthy."

When we rationalize away our decision, we can feel good about eating what we want.

In contrast, we find it much more difficult to conjure up powerful reasons for avoiding junk food:

- "I have real food waiting for me to enjoy at home."
- "I want my waistline to stay exactly where it is."
- "I'd rather eat food that truly satisfies and nourishes my body."
- "I value my health over momentary pleasures."

- "I only put high-quality fuels into this highly complex, finely-tuned machine."
- "I don't want to become addicted to foods that are full of fat, sugar, and salt that artificially overstimulate the pleasure centers of my brain and promote compulsive eating that leads to obesity and disease."
- "I only put molecules into my body that are good for it and give it exactly what it needs to function, thrive, repair itself, and fight off disease."
- "I don't eat Frankenfoods [to use Dr. Joel Fuhrman's term]."
- "I want to wake up tomorrow with no regrets."

So, stop salivating over junk food. Instead, quickly turn your eyes away from junk-food temptations, engage your frontal cortex, and remember all the reasons why you should avoid it. Don't give in to "the pleasure trap."

Are you conscious of just how vulnerable your body is?

Sometimes it seems like we are not very aware of just how vulnerable our bodies are to physical insult, injury, pain, discomfort, and even death. It's almost as if we are surrounded by a protective psychological bubble that maintains a certain illusion of invincibility. When we are feeling good physically, we downplay just how easily we can be injured. However, anyone who has visited their local emergency room or physical therapy department has seen a far different reality. There, emergency room doctors frantically try to save lives and stitch people back together and physical therapists try to help patients painfully regain even simple movements of their body and limbs.

Our bodies are tender flesh and bone and as such are subject to a whole host of physical threats. Some of these threats are overtly physical, such as those resulting from skiing mishaps, workplace injuries, and automobile accidents. Others are the result of environmental conditions, such as not having clean air, pure water, sufficient food, sanitary living conditions, or ambient temperatures that fall within a very narrow range. Others are the result of natural disasters or criminal acts that cause severe injury and death. And other threats are from viruses, bacteria, parasites, toxins, carcinogens, and toxic junk food that can destroy our health and kill or disable us quickly or slowly from the inside out.

Many of us think of our body as our friend—like someone who would never turn on us—but our body, when subject to these threats, can very quickly become an instrument of severe pain and torture. Sadly, we don't fully appreciate this fact until we are the ones who are suffering. Only then do we fully appreciate how quickly and completely our reality can change from one moment to the next.

Because of these threats, we are cautioned to take protective measures, such as fastening our seat belts, wearing a bike helmet, staying out of high crime areas, avoiding undue risk, and anticipating accidents before they happen. No one questions the importance of taking such sensible measures.

But when it comes to our health, how many of us see our bodies as just as vulnerable to *dietary* threats? How many of us, for example, think it does not matter what we feed our bodies or that our bodies can take whatever we dish out to them and still stay strong and healthy and not turn on us?

If so, then deflate the psychological bubble of invulnerability that prevents you from seeing reality and recognize that your body is just as vulnerable to nutritional abuse as it is to other threats. Keep your body as your friend and avoid turning it into an instrument of pain or torture because of your own dietary choices by feeding it only whole, plant-based foods.

How "getting to healthy" will help you in other areas of your life

The skills and character attributes you have acquired in getting to healthy will not only benefit your health—they will benefit you in other areas of your life as well. For example, in getting to healthy, you have learned:

- Self-discipline—to control what you eat and do not eat and to care for your body—which will boost your self-esteem, your self-confidence, and your sense of accomplishment and will readily transfer to other areas of your life that require self-discipline,
- Not to rely on emotional crutches as substitutes for personal growth,
- Not to make excuses or rationalize away your behavior,
- That actions and decisions have immediate and long-term consequences—for good or bad,

- That life is full of cause-and-effect relationships that play out even if you are ignorant of them, deny them, or ignore them,
- That self-education, preparation, and social support structures are important keys to achieving success,
- That self-encouragement, patience, and long-suffering is a better strategy for self-improvement then self-hatred and self-condemnation,
- To recognize that dangers exist in life and how to avoid them,
- To take a long-term perspective in making decisions,
- To judge others and their ideas more carefully and thoughtfully, and
- To love happiness, personal freedom, and conformance to truth.

Surely these are skills and attributes that will bless your life, not just your health. Getting to healthy is not just about eating better. It promotes personal growth and achievement.

PART 3.

CONCLUSION

Congratulations on getting to healthy! You have accomplished a difficult and great task in your life—one that will reap many amazing benefits.

In reflection, you have spent the last 21 weeks getting to healthy. You are probably eating more healthily now than 95 percent of Americans. You have made it through the painful "withdrawal" phase and are no longer addicted to unhealthy "Frankenfoods." You eat more whole fruits, grains, vegetables, legumes, nuts, and seeds. You naturally prefer to eat healthy, nutrient-dense foods over unhealthy foods full of fat, sugar, and salt. You avoid animal products, junk foods, fast foods, and processed foods. You have developed a great respect for your body, are highly disciplined, and take pride in taking care of yourself.

As a result, you are enjoying the incredible benefits of healthy eating. You feel younger, are in better health, and have more vitality than ever before. Some of your previous health problems have probably diminished or even disappeared. You probably shed some excess pounds, which you have easily kept off. Your annual physical returned some amazing blood test results. In short, you have witnessed for yourself the cause-and-effect relationship between how you eat, how you feel, and good health.

Now it is your turn to pay it forward by helping others understand this relationship, by encouraging them to make the transition to healthy, and by supporting them through the process. "Others" include your children, your spouse, your grandchildren, your parents, your friends, your neighbors, and your co-workers. Because you care about them, you want them to avoid unnecessary disease, pain, and suffering in their lives and to live the healthiest, most fulfilling lives possible.

You know they need their health to do this. *They* probably don't fully appreciate that fact yet. Your job is to help them acquire that understanding and then to live by it.

Don't let them down.

ABOUT THE AUTHOR

John S Hoffman, Ph.D., learned about healthy eating and the relationship between diet, health, and disease avoidance only after he was diagnosed with two forms of deadly cancer within a two-week period. After overcoming cancer, he subsequently made the transition to healthy eating and now seeks to help others do the same. Dr. Hoffman has a doctorate in instructional science and a bachelor's degree in psychology. He is the author of *The Emotional Foundations of Loving Relationships* and two other professional books.

Made in the USA
Middletown, DE
28 August 2021